THE
FLAVOR
POINT
DIET

THE DELICIOUS, BREAKTHROUGH PLAN TO
TURN OFF YOUR HUNGER AND
LOSE THE WEIGHT FOR GOOD

DAVID L. KATZ, MD, MPH,
Director of the Yale Prevention Research Center

with CATHERINE S. KATZ, PhD

RODALE

Book design by Christina Gaugler
Photograph on page 295 by Justin Appi

Library of Congress Cataloging-in-Publication Data

Katz, David L., MD
    The flavor point diet : the delicious, breakthrough plan to turn off your hunger and lose the weight for good / David L. Katz with Catherine S. Katz.
        p.   cm.
    Includes bibliographical references and index.
    ISBN-13 978–1–59486–162–8 hardcover
    ISBN-10 1–59486–162–5 hardcover
    1. Reducing diets.   2. Weight loss.   I. Katz, Catherine S.   II. Title.
RM222.2.K363   2006
613.2'5—dc22   2005025985

Distributed to the trade by Holtzbrinck Publishers

2   4   6   8   10   9   7   5   3   1   hardcover

"Written by one of the most knowledgeable nutrition experts I know, this book uses the science on the biology and psychology of flavors to offer up one good idea after another for optimal eating."

—Kelly D. Brownell, PhD, chair and professor of psychology, professor of epidemiology and public health, and director of the Rudd Center for Food Policy & Obesity at Yale University

"*The Flavor Point Diet* is a science-based real-life (and real simple) program written with the consumer in mind. It makes sense that our sensory overload extends from video and television screens to the table, but when people perceive weight loss as work, it's difficult to achieve. Dr. Katz respects the temptations that surround us, but he shows you how to 'get your house in order' and get on the weight-loss track.

"Allow yourself to be guided by the caring Dr. Katz. *The Flavor Point Diet* is nutritionally balanced, full of ideas for easy meals and snacks, with great recipes plus information about shopping, reading food labels, dining out in restaurants, plus good advice for making healthy choices wherever you go. This is a fun program to follow . . . you can achieve your weight goal without dieting or deprivation."

—Susan Burke, MS, RD, LD/N, CDE, vice president of nutrition services at eDiets.com

"Dr. David Katz is America's 'Go-to Guy' when it comes to a sensible, sane, and science-based approach to personal health. That's why you see him on ABC's *Good Morning America* and why I asked him to help steer the effort to promote health in all 50 states through the National Governors Association. A brilliant and respected researcher, he's also a highly experienced medical practitioner whose clear and earthy communicative style make him fun to read. He's a doc that will keep you in stitches—the right way!"

—Mike Huckabee, governor of Arkansas, chairman of the National Governors Association, and author of *Quit Digging Your Grave with a Knife and Fork*

"There's nothing more confusing than walking down the aisle of a grocery store. With Dr. Katz at your side, you'll always make the right choices. *The Flavor Point Diet* is a terrific achievement, blending science, insight, and the kind of real-world guidance we all need. I recommend it highly."

—David Zinczenko, editor-in-chief, *Men's Health* magazine

"Dr. Katz is an unfailing source of first-rate, scientifically based advice about good nutrition and the steps that need to be taken for achieving a healthy weight. This book contains a road map for all of us—no matter our age."

—Francine Kaufman, MD, president of the American Diabetes Association

On behalf of my family—Rebecca, Corinda, Valerie, Natalia, and Gabriel; Catherine and myself—I dedicate *The Flavor Point Diet* to your family. Because in unity there is strength. Because weight loss and lasting weight control should come about through the pursuit of health—and health should be a family affair. So here's to you, your success, and good health—and the same for those who love you and share your journey.

CONTENTS

*Tapping into the Flavor Point will revolutionize the way
you think about eating.*

PART 1: THE SCIENCE

*Until now, your brain has controlled your food choices.
Soon, your food choices will control your brain!*

*Although many variables influence how much you eat,
flavor matters most.*

Fill up on fewer calories in three easy steps.

PART 2: THE PLAN

*6 weeks of delicious, convenient, and flavor-friendly meals
that turn down the Flavor Point.*

*More than 100 options that are so delicious, you won't believe
they're this good for you.*

*You've graduated from the school of flavor themes. You no longer
need them as long as you adhere to the Flavor Point principles.*

ACKNOWLEDGMENTS

While two people can conceive a baby, and one person alone can bear and deliver that baby, it has been said it takes a village to enable that baby to develop, mature, and thrive. This is true of books as well.

I may take much personal credit (or blame, should any see it that way) for the concept of *The Flavor Point Diet*. And certainly, I have labored over its embryonic development for years. (The gestational period of books is longer than that of people!) But for inspiring the concept in the first place, refining it, maturing it, and taking something as ephemeral as an idea and turning it into something as tangible as a book, I have depended on, and owe thanks to, a veritable village full of colleagues.

The first of these I want to acknowledge is my literary agent, Rick Broadhead. Rick is thoughtful and wise, careful and meticulous, enthusiastic and supportive, practical and candid. He has been the ideal agent and has become a friend. I am very pleased to have found him (or vice versa) before he becomes too busy and successful to have time for me! To any aspiring authors out there—this guy's the best!

I am grateful to Mariska van Aalst, my editor at Rodale, for seeing more in my book proposal than was actually there; for helping me identify the book I was looking to write; and for her faith that I could then write it! Mariska really has been more than the book's editor—she has been a confidante, friend, and trusted advisor at every step of its development. All this while having a baby (of the human variety). So my heartfelt thanks to Mariska for her vision and support, along with my congratulations to her and her family.

I owe special thanks to Alisa Bauman, who stepped in while Mariska was out on maternity leave. If I and my book were a baton, Alisa took hold in a smooth pass and then went on to run a magnificent leg of this relay race. A great deal that is good in the book is directly thanks to Alisa, who edited every line with a masterful eye for clarity. Any line or passage that is less good or unclear than it should be is doubtless something Alisa tried unsuccessfully to talk me out of!

I am grateful to Sumiya Khan, MS, RD, and Dina Aronson, MS, RD, for their invaluable contribution of nutritional analyses. I am proud that *The Flavor Point Diet* conforms to the very highest standards of nutrition throughout, and it's thanks to Sumiya and Dina that I can say that with confidence and back it up with data. To Dina, I add thanks, on behalf of Catherine especially, for becoming a genuine and much-relied-upon partner in this venture. We simply couldn't have done it without you. Thanks!

I am indebted to the many nutrition professionals from whom I have learned so much throughout my career and who conducted the research upon which *The Flavor Point Diet* is based. First and foremost, I thank Barbara Rolls, PhD, of Penn State University. Professor Rolls is a true luminary in the fields of appetite and weight regulation. Her research over years and decades is an eloquent and elegant demonstration of the power of science to confront and overcome challenges in human health. Much of what we all know about appetite and its control is thanks to the prolific work of Professor Rolls.

I thank Professor Linda Bartoshuk, my Yale colleague and one of the world's leading authorities on taste perception, for inspiring my interest in the power of food flavor over appetite—and for directing me to the work of Professor Rolls many years ago. I acknowledge, as well, but will not name for fear of unpardonable omissions, the many colleagues, mentors, teachers, friends, and predecessors who have enriched the field of nutrition and weight control with their contributions. In any effort to reach a new height or attain a new vista, we stand on the shoulders of others. I thank you all for holding me up.

Special thanks to the 20 participants in our pilot test of the Flavor Point Diet. You'll hear from them throughout the book—but here, I want them to hear from me. I am indebted to you all. I extend my appreciation to Michelle Larovera, and Dr. Zubaida Faridi, of the Yale Prevention Research Center, who managed the pilot test with such grace, good cheer, and professionalism.

My wife, Catherine, ever my partner, best friend, best editor, harshest critic, and staunchest supporter, is my collaborating author. I cannot hope to thank her as she deserves. She has taken my theories of nutrition and translated them into a delightful, delicious, real-world practicality. She did that first for the fortunate members of the Katz household. She does that now for you. We can both be grateful to her for that. I, of course, owe her far more, for she fills my life with joy and love and meaning every day.

On behalf of Catherine, as well as myself, I offer thanks to our children: Rebecca, Corinda, Valerie, Natalia, and Gabriel. They helped in the kitchen and taste-tested the many Flavor Point trials—and occasional Flavor Point errors! And they did it all with good cheer, esprit de corps, and enthusiasm. But more importantly, these terrific kids turned over both of their parents to the care and nurturing of a book for many months. While this didn't quite turn them into orphans, it certainly did come at a cost to them. If they ever complained about that cost, I can't recall. So thanks, gang—we love you! And we have some together time to make up to you!

Thanks as well to my parents, Susan and Don Katz, for their never-wavering faith and support—and their timely attention to our children! They are the likely reason *Flavor Point* did not induce more disgruntlement among the Katz kids.

On behalf of this collaborating village, I am proud to present *The Flavor Point Diet*. All members deserve credit for its merits and whatever good it accomplishes. But should any omissions, deficiencies, errors, or misstatements be discerned, responsibility for them resides with me.

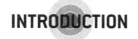

MIND OVER APPETITE

Tapping into the Flavor Point will revolutionize the way you think about eating.

At some point during every eating experience, we all begin to feel full and *fulfilled*. When you reach that point of fulfillment—what I call the *Flavor Point*—you stop eating. If you reach the Flavor Point early enough, you will feel full and fulfilled on fewer calories. If you reach the Flavor Point too late, you overeat.

How do you reach the Flavor Point more quickly and fill up on fewer calories?

That's what the Flavor Point Diet is all about. This revolutionary diet taps into this little-known but scientifically proven fact: Flavor variety stimulates the appetite center in your brain, while flavor repetition soothes it. You can eat a variety of flavors over time, but eating too many flavors at any *one* time puts your brain's appetite center into overdrive.

Let that sink in for a minute. It's every bit as profound, powerful, and life changing as it is simple. To safely and permanently lose weight without being hungry, you need only organize the flavors in your meals and snacks. Don't misunderstand me, though. You don't need to give up flavors. You don't need to give up specific foods or entire categories of foods. You don't need to give up the joy of eating delicious food, and you certainly don't need to give up the convenience of easy-to-prepare foods.

THE POWER OF FLAVOR ORGANIZATION

From breakfast cereals to snack foods to fast foods, our culinary land-scape has become crowded with an overabundance of conflicting flavors that overstimulate important appetite-controlling cells in our brains, making us need more and more food to reach the Flavor Point. For example, many sweet breakfast cereals contain as much salt as potato chips. Yes, salt! Conversely, salty snack foods often include lots of sugar. You don't always notice all of these flavors when you eat, but your brain registers their presence, triggering hunger and overeating.

When you taste too many flavors at once—whether from too many different foods or too many flavors processed into one food—you overeat before feeling full. On the other hand, when you organize flavors in your diet, you feel full and satisfied on fewer calories and lose weight *without feeling hungry!* Quite simply, you will *want* to eat less!

The Flavor Point Diet subdues appetite on two levels. First, it uses the powerful benefits of flavor themes to subtly organize your eating. These themes infuse your meals with a specific flavor, such as orange or chocolate or pineapple. When you taste this flavor repeatedly throughout your day, you more quickly satisfy your brain's appetite center so you're able to fill up on fewer calories. Second, you'll shift to a new way of eating—to the Flavor Point way of eating. You'll learn how to choose and cook delicious meals using relatively simple, wholesome, minimally processed foods that don't contain an overabundance of extraneous flavors.

Over the next 6 weeks and beyond, the Flavor Point Diet will change your appetite, your weight, your appearance, your health, your relationship with food, and your life—for good! The plan comprises three phases.

Phase 1. During the first 4 weeks of the meal plan, you'll drape a delicate flavor theme over your meals for an entire day, with every meal and snack sharing a common ingredient. On Cranberry Day, for example, you'll eat delicious cranberry-banana muffins for breakfast, a salad with cranberries for lunch, cranberry and onion turkey cutlets for dinner, and Cranberry-Vanilla Soft Ice Cream for dessert. On Pineapple Day, you'll have a pineapple smoothie for breakfast, Pineapple-Walnut Chicken Salad for lunch, and Pineapple Shrimp for dinner. On Lemon Day, you'll have lemon-poppy muffins for breakfast, Lemon Tabbouleh Salad for lunch, and lemon-flavored tilapia for dinner.

This subtle yet repeated exposure to the same flavors will subdue your ap-

FLAVOR FLUENCY

SENSORY-SPECIFIC SATIETY: The tendency to feel full and stop eating when flavors are limited and to stay hungry and keep eating when flavors are diverse.

petite center in a delicious and powerful way. But you won't eat enough of the flavor of the day for it to feel monotonous. Instead, your appetite center will merely register the flavor and, as a result, feel soothed and contented.

Phase 2. As you get into the habit of choosing and preparing foods according to Flavor Point principles, you won't need to depend on the daily flavor themes as much to control your appetite. In other words, as your mastery increases, you'll need fewer rules. This is why, during weeks 5 and 6, the meal plan includes a greater variety of daily flavors. In this phase, each meal or snack has a theme, but there's no single theme throughout the day. Thus, the flavor theme for your breakfast will not be the same as the one for your lunch, and each of those will differ from dinner. For instance, breakfast might have a lemon theme, lunch a basil theme, and dinner a tomato theme. In each meal, the flavors are subtle but effective, harmonizing the food—and your appetite!

Phase 3. The Flavor Point Meal Plan guides you through 6 weeks of weight loss by using flavor themes for each day during the first 4 weeks and then for each meal during weeks 5 and 6. After that, you'll be ready for phase 3—the beginning of the rest of your life! Phase 3 is permanent, using flavor management at the level of individual foods. We provide examples to get you launched, but then, with the habits you've acquired, the knowledge you've gained, and the principles you've mastered, you'll be ready for lifelong Flavor Point success. During phase 3, you'll continue to lose weight until you reach your goal, and then you'll keep it off.

In Chapter 6, you'll find dozens of tips to help you convert your old family recipes into meals that are just as delicious but conform to Flavor Point principles. In the appendix, you'll find lots of Flavor Point Diet–approved brands of simply flavored, delicious, and convenient foods sold at your local supermarket.

From the first day to the last on the meal plan, you will consume a perfectly balanced, healthful diet. You could stay on any phase of the meal plan forever—it's that good for you. As a physician, preventive medicine specialist, and parent, I wouldn't have it any other way. I am not a "diet doctor"; I am a doctor who happens to be an expert on diet and nutrition. No matter how important weight loss may be to you, your overall health—and that of your family—is what matters most to me.

DOES THIS REALLY WORK?

As I was putting the finishing touches on this book, many people asked me, somewhat skeptically, "Can flavor themes really subdue appetite?" Am I proposing something radical? Inventing a theory? Going out on a limb? Defying my academic colleagues? Not at all.

Under the scientific-sounding name *sensory-specific satiety,* the Flavor Point's main concept has been appearing in the scientific literature for nearly 3 decades. It has been percolating near the surface of dietary guidance, but its full potential for weight control simply wasn't recognized—until now. Although this meal plan is unique, the science is tried and true.

In Chapter 1, you'll learn how millions of years of evolution have hardwired this trait into the appetite center of the brain of every human on the planet. If you've ever overeaten, however, you may already understand how it works. Have you ever enjoyed a delicious holiday feast and eaten until you felt stuffed? Did each bite taste slightly less delicious than the bite before, especially as you became more and more full? Did the main course eventually completely lose its appeal? At some point, did you put your hand on your stomach and groan, "I'm so full I couldn't eat another bite!" And in the next breath ask, "What's for dessert?"

Yep, you found room for dessert, didn't you? Me, too! It wasn't because of that hollow leg or extra stomach that some wisecracking relative referred to. It was because of sensory-specific satiety! You had filled up on the savory flavors provided by the main dishes but not on the sweet flavor of dessert.

As you'll soon learn, each flavor we eat stimulates a different set of cells in the brain. Sweet flavors stimulate one area of the brain's appetite center, salty another, and sour yet another. Once you turn on an area of the appetite center, you must eat until those cells register fullness. If you turn on many areas at once, you must eat much more food before you feel full. Turn on just one or two areas, and you'll eat less but feel just as satisfied.

I owe a lot to the scientists who have studied sensory-specific satiety during the past several decades. As soon as I learned about it, the power of it was immediately obvious, and I began applying it to my diet and those of my patients. Although many scientists have documented this phenomenon over the years, the Flavor Point Diet is the first to use sensory-specific satiety to enable long-term weight control without hunger.

In my work at Yale as well as in my private practice, I've now counseled hundreds of patients who desperately wanted to lose weight. When they came to me, most of them knew what they needed to do to shed pounds. They knew they should eat less and exercise more, but they couldn't figure out how to do it. Each time they went on a diet, they lost some weight. Eventually, though, their cravings and hunger would win out, they'd break the diet, and they'd gain the weight back—and usually more.

When I taught these patients about sensory-specific satiety and how to use Flavor Point principles to subdue appetite, weight management without hunger suddenly became feasible for them. They would tell me that for the first time in their lives, they had no difficulty holding themselves to reasonable portions. They finally were able to enjoy eating without guilt. It changed their lives and those of their families. I observed this over and over, using each experience to refine the Flavor Point plan—and here you have the culmination of that work.

Recently, I asked 20 men and women to test the meal plan you'll find in this book. Some wanted to lose just a few pounds; others wanted to lose many more. They came from all walks of life and included stay-at-home moms, working mothers and fathers, and singles. Most shared one trait: They were busy and didn't have time for complicated meal preparation.

Their results, after 12 weeks on the plan, just blew me away. On average, they lost over 16 pounds. (One gentleman lost 31 pounds!) Their blood cholesterol levels dropped an average of 14 points. Blood pressure, blood sugar, and other health indicators also improved. They lost an average of 3½ inches off their waists! Not only did their clothes fit better but they also felt more energetic, slept better at night, and experienced fewer cravings. Most important, they *loved* the food—and so did their spouses and children, who in many cases also lost weight and improved their health. Officially, they weren't even on the diet!

The study participants told me that their cravings for certain foods shifted. After 12 weeks, even the most hard-core junk-food junkies among them preferred this new way of eating. Take a look at some of their comments.

- "I'm full and definitely satisfied on this program. I had a little bit of dessert the other night—and that's all I wanted. It actually tasted too sweet!"

FLAVOR FLUENCY

THE FLAVOR POINT: The point when the flavors in your food fill up the appetite center in your brain, subduing hunger and appetite. In the part of the brain called the hypothalamus, each of us has a number of specialized cells that respond to flavor. Think of those cells as a series of meters, measuring from empty to full. Each meter responds to a particular taste, from sweet to sour, salty to savory, and everything in between. Whenever you turn on an appetite meter, it must register fullness before it turns off again. The fewer meters you turn on, the less you eat before you feel full and satisfied—and the sooner you reach the Flavor Point.

- "Not only are the foods delicious, but I don't have heartburn anymore!"
- "I actually look forward to eating dinner every night. The food is excellent. I love this program, and I think I could eat like this forever."

Those study participants followed an extended 12-week version of the Flavor Point plan. I've streamlined it for you. In this book, you'll find 6 weeks' worth of mouthwatering, simple, convenient, appetite-subduing meals. These meals have helped me, my family, my friends, and my patients fill up on fewer calories—enjoying food as well as the satisfaction of lasting weight control. Now they will do the same for you!

(continued on page xxii)

Results from the Flavor Point

Our group of testers, 20 in all, tried the Flavor Point Diet for 12 weeks, and their results were amazing. Not only did they lose pounds and inches, feel more energetic, and experience fewer cravings, several key measures of their health improved dramatically. Check out some stats from the Flavor Point.

	AVERAGE	MOST CHANGED
Pounds lost:	16.7	31
Change in BMI:	−2.7	−4.2
Inches off of waist:	3.53	7
Percent body fat lost:	4.82	8
Blood pressure points dropped:	11.4	28
Reduction in resting heart rate (beats per minute):	4.86	12
Total points cholesterol lowered:	14.2	72
Fasting blood glucose (mg/Dl):	−1.13	−15

Satisfaction at the Flavor Point

THE FLAVOR FACTS

Name: Debbie Vashlishan

Age: 50

Hometown: Oxford, Connecticut

Family status: Married with two children, ages 24 and 25

Occupation: Registered nurse

Starting weight: 201

Pounds lost: 17 in 12 weeks

Health stats: Blood pressure dropped 16 points; resting heart rate improved; waist measurement shrank $3\frac{1}{2}$ inches; 5 percent decline in body fat

"I gained weight slowly and steadily over the years. It eventually crept up to about 200 pounds. I knew I needed to make a lifestyle change, so when I heard a few women discussing Dr. Katz's new program, I was intrigued and decided to go for it. I was thrilled when I heard I'd been chosen.

"My husband has been doing the program with me, and he actually lost more weight than I did in the first 12 weeks—24 pounds! More important, he's been able to cut his blood pressure medication dosage in half.

"Health improvements aside, we're eating good, healthful foods— and they taste great! I'm discovering many new seasonings, like curry, that I really enjoy. Also, many of the vinegars and oils the plan recommends add wonderful flavor to the recipes. I don't feel hungry on this program, and my cravings are gone. When I first heard about the flavor themes, I thought, 'We're going to eat apples for a whole day? Eww!' Eventually, I realized the other foods mixed in with the theme of the day, like nuts and chicken, keep you from getting sick of it. The concept really works.

"Both my husband and I love the recipes. I have actually served some of the dishes to guests because they're so tasty. On my days off, I make the French toast, muffins, or multigrain pancakes with honey yogurt sauce for breakfast. The Pumpkin and Chocolate Grilled Panini is one of my favorite lunch recipes, as well as the peanut butter and peach jam sandwich. I had the sandwich on Easter Sunday—I made it and took it to work, and I couldn't wait to go to lunch to have that sandwich!

"For dinner, the pastas are great, and my daughter loves the chicken in Dijon 'creamy' mushroom sauce. My husband and I aren't big fish eaters, but we like the tilapia, so we substitute that for tuna and salmon, and it works just fine.

"For a snack, the fruit smoothies are both refreshing and filling. I also like the granola. We went hiking with another couple the other day, and I made individual baggies of granola with nuts and apricots. It was plenty to get us all through the hike.

"The main dishes and snacks are satisfying enough, but there are also a bunch of good desserts on the program. We love Baked Bananas with Rum-Pecan Topping, amaretto strawberry salad, brownies, and Peach Flat Cake. And who ever heard of indulgence days on a diet? I've done the chocolate day twice, and I plan to try the coconut day in the future.

"I've also learned some handy tricks I'll take with me forever. I now use olive oil on veggies instead of butter or cheese. Instead of spreading mayonnaise on a sandwich, I use hummus. I also carry a container of powdered milk in my purse wherever I go to use in my coffee.

"It feels wonderful to have so many people tell me I look good and that my face looks thinner. My clothes fit better, I have much more energy, and it's a little weird, but I've also noticed that my fingernails are stronger. Both my husband and I love Dr. Katz's program and are going to stick with it indefinitely." ▪

DELICIOUS AND EFFECTIVE

In this diet, the pleasures of eating food that's good and food that's good for you can—and do—come together. The joys of food and of lasting weight control and good health are not mutually exclusive! When you commit to the Flavor Point Diet, you commit to a diet that:

Delivers lasting weight loss. Based on the results of the people who tested the Flavor Point Diet before this book went to press, you can expect to lose 9 to 16 pounds in 6 weeks and continue losing weight until you reach your goal. The Flavor Point Diet isn't one that you go on and off of. Rather, it provides a simple and easy transition to a new way of choosing and organizing foods—forever.

Not only helps you shed fat but also improves your health. Every step of the way, the pattern of foods and nutrients you will consume is as good or better than the recommendations of the U.S. Department of Health and Human Services, the Institute of Medicine, the American Heart Association, the American Cancer Society, the American Diabetes Association, and the American Dietetic Association.

Liberates you from the bondage of shunning certain so-called fattening foods. At no point does this diet restrict any foods. At no point does it place a whole nutrient category off-limits. Because the Flavor Point Diet is not based on food exclusions—that's right, there are *none*—each phase of the plan is balanced, sane, delicious, healthful, and in step with the very best of modern nutrition science.

Allows you and your entire family to lose weight together. Unlike so many diets out there, the Flavor Point Diet is safe for your whole family. Yes, your kids can follow it with you. Yes, it's safe during pregnancy. Yes, it's fine while breastfeeding. Yes, it's appropriate if you have diabetes. Yes, anyone can follow this diet at any time! It is safe for life.

Makes healthful eating quick and easy. The Flavor Point Diet replaces the convenient processed and fast foods that trigger overeating with foods that trigger fullness and are just as convenient and delicious. Many breakfasts and lunches in the Flavor Point Meal Plan take 5 minutes or less to prepare! Many dinners take 15 minutes or less.

Puts the joy back into eating. The Flavor Point Meal Plan includes incredibly delicious meals, snacks, and desserts. In fact, you can eat dessert every night if you are so inclined!

Flavor management makes all this possible. You're about to embark on an exciting journey to a slimmer, healthier you. In Chapters 1 and 2, you'll discover the science behind the meal plan. In Chapter 3, you'll find out how the meal plan works. Chapters 4 and 5 bring you the Flavor Point Meal Plan and corresponding recipes. Finally, in Chapter 6, you'll find out how to move on to phase 3 and maintain the Flavor Point way of eating for life.

Since the food is delicious and the nutrition stellar every step of the way, why would you ever go off this plan? If, after 6 weeks, you find that you have lost a lot of weight (you will), are feeling great (you'll see), and are loving the food (just wait!)—why on Earth would you ever look back? You won't. The next 6 weeks and beyond will change your whole relationship with food, and your body, forever.

PART 1

THE SCIENCE

MEET YOUR APPETITE CENTER

Until now, your brain has controlled your food choices. Soon, your food choices will control your brain!

Study after study points to this indisputable but little-known fact: the more foods and flavors we humans taste, the more we must eat to feel satisfied. The fewer foods and flavors we taste, the less we eat and the more satisfied we feel on fewer calories.

We are, quite simply, hardwired to want variety in our diets. We're hardwired to get fed up with eating the same food again and again. We're hardwired to rediscover hunger when some new flavor opportunity comes along.

This hardwiring, however, doesn't require that we all suffer a boring culinary existence in order to remain slim. No, you don't need to eat the same food over and over again—although that tactic certainly would work. Rather, by using the science of sensory-specific satiety to your advantage, you can enjoy delicious meals and still lose weight without hunger! The Flavor Point Diet will show you how. You will consume a variety of flavors over time, just not an excessive variety all at one time!

Once you understand how to use this concept to your advantage, you can lower your Flavor Point—the point at which you feel satisfied and stop eating—and automatically eat less and lose weight. Once you do, you'll never again find yourself out of control, mindlessly shoveling forkful after forkful of food into your mouth.

WHY WE OVEREAT

The most important, prevalent, and powerful reason we eat and overeat is sensory delight: We do it because we see, smell, and taste food. You, along with every other human, have a sensory relay system that connects your mouth to your brain, your brain to your stomach, and your stomach back to your brain. Ultimately, your brain is in charge of your eating behavior. It controls what you eat and what you like to eat. As soon as you taste food, the sensory information registers in the hypothalamus in the brain, which, depending on the flavor of the food, sends out signals to eat more or eat less. Because of this sensory relay system, the appetite center in your hypothalamus can become aroused—and in some cases overly aroused—by how a food tastes.

If you can reach the Flavor Point with fewer calories, you can feel just as full and satisfied but also be thinner! Getting your brain to tell your mind, and your mouth, "That will do; I'm satisfied" with fewer calories is what the Flavor Point Diet is all about.

To learn how to work with your appetite center, you must first understand it. It's time for you and your brain to become better acquainted.

As soon as you bite into any food, sensory stimulation of nerve endings on the tongue leads to the release of a number of chemicals, including opioids, into the bloodstream. You release more opioids—the body's natural versions of drugs like morphine—when you consume foods high in sugar and fat, creating a powerful, neurochemical drive to overeat those foods. These opioids and other chemicals enter the bloodstream and carry their messages to the hypothalamus, which sends out yet another set of chemicals to regulate appetite. The more flavors your taste buds register, the more stimulated the hypothalamus becomes, releasing the hunger-promoting hormone neuropeptide Y. When you taste a lot of flavors at once, the brain releases a lot of neuropeptide Y.

Meanwhile, in response to the smell and taste of food, your stomach produces the hormone ghrelin, which also stimulates appetite. It continues to produce this hormone until you eat enough food to literally fill your stomach and stretch the stomach wall. Farther down the line, in your intestines, levels of several hormones rise to varying degrees—depending on the nature of your meal—either inducing more hunger or turning off hunger.

To understand how your food choices can influence this complex chain of events, let's take a closer look at how this all works by comparing the neurochemical response to two foods you might eat for breakfast: a sausage, egg, and cheese English muffin sandwich and a bowl of oatmeal.

FLAVOR FLUENCY

SATIATION: The point at which you feel full, stop eating, and push back from the table. *Satiety* is the state of feeling full and satisfied.

In the mouth: The mix of sugar, fat, and salt in the egg sandwich triggers the release of more opioids than the oatmeal does. These opioids create a powerful, neurochemical drive to eat more sandwich.

In the brain: The sandwich's sausage, cheese, and muffin offer many varied tastes, causing neuropeptide Y—and hunger—to surge. The simple flavors of the oatmeal result in the release of much less neuropeptide Y.

In the stomach: The sandwich delivers a lot of calories in a small package. It doesn't stimulate the stomach's stretch receptors nearly as quickly as the oatmeal, allowing ghrelin levels to remain high long after you've overeaten. You must eat many more egg sandwich calories than oatmeal calories before the stomach wall registers fullness.

In the intestines: The highly processed sandwich bread less effectively suppresses hunger-producing hormones than does the oatmeal, again leaving you feeling hungry despite the abundance of calories.

(continued on page 8)

Satisfaction at the Flavor Point

THE FLAVOR FACTS

Name: Lisa Seaberg

Age: 30

Hometown: Ansonia, Connecticut

Family status: Single

Occupation: Communication
    specialist

Starting weight: 163

Pounds lost: 12 in 12 weeks

Health stats: Blood pressure
    dropped 15 points; cholesterol
    dropped 9 points; waist mea-
    surement shrank 2 inches;
    8 percent decline in body fat

"I was never obese, but I come from a family of fat people, and I was well on my way to becoming heavy myself. During the past 3 to 4 years, I gained 20 pounds. I had already read Dr. Katz's first book and found it offered some great advice, so I decided to try his program.

"Before I started, my diet wasn't terrible, but it was unbalanced. I usually ate a decent breakfast (oatmeal and coffee). For lunch, however, I ate whatever the cafeteria was serving, whether it was chicken or macaroni and cheese. Sometimes I would skip dinner and just have a bowl of cereal or an egg, or I would buy dinner out. I live by myself, so it didn't seem worth it for me to cook a whole meal. Being a big chocoholic, I ate a candy bar every day after lunch.

"Dr. Katz's program has not only taught me how to cook well for myself, it has also taught me to enjoy doing it. I actually shocked all my friends because I was notorious for not cooking (I actually used my oven for a storage space for a while). Now I'm totally comfortable with cooking. I actually find it fun!

"On most days, I stick to the meal plan for breakfast, lunch, and dinner because I really like trying the new dishes. I try to swap the days so I can have the omelets or pancakes on the weekend (they are my favorites for breakfast). For lunch, I love the different variations of the spinach-lentil salads, but my favorite is the dill chicken salad. For dinner, the shrimp pasta primavera is the one I keep going back to the most.

"Snack-wise, I tend to go for the fresh fruit most often, but I also enjoy the oat bran pretzels. I never cared much for pretzels before, but these are quite good.

"One of the best parts is that even though I'm losing weight, I feel like I'm eating more food than ever before. I always liked healthful foods (for instance, I was already eating whole wheat pasta), but I didn't know how to incorporate them into my diet in a realistic way. Now I do.

"The most surprising change? I haven't craved the chocolate after lunch. I have to admit I was happy to see the chocolate day on the menu, but I haven't had the urge to break down and have a candy bar!

"Not only have I changed my eating habits with this program, I've also made a concerted effort to become more active. I joined the YMCA for the fitness facilities, and I go inline skating and take karate classes. I also rescued my bike from beneath a pile of wood in my mom's garage. I feel like it doesn't make sense to change the way I eat without changing my activity level as well.

"And it's all paying off. I feel so much better physically and mentally. I have more energy and a greater sense of well-being, and I'm no longer falling asleep at my desk at 3 or 4 in the afternoon. Other people have noticed the change in me. One of my coworkers said my face was getting thinner, and I guess it inspired her. She came in to work the next day and said she had exercised after work because she was motivated by how good I look!

"Even though I've finished my initial 12 weeks, I've been sticking with the program and planning what I'm going to eat every day (so I don't get hungry and decide to order a pizza). The structure is a good thing for me, especially because I love the foods! And because Dr. Katz's program is working so well, I've been talking it up a lot. I would recommend it to anyone. Thanks, Dr. Katz!"

Flavor Pointer

TASTE TRIGGERS AND THE FOOD INDUSTRY'S SMOKING GUN

The food industry puts sugar, salt, and fat—all potent appetite stimulators—to very good use. Humans prefer sweet tastes from birth, which is why the industry processes sugar, with a variety of often misleading names (such as high-fructose corn syrup), into most packaged foods. Don't expect a food with added sugar to taste sweet, though. Just enough sugar is added to trigger your appetite but not quite enough for you to notice that your chips are sweet as well as salty.

You'll also find salt in most processed foods. Sweet foods, such as desserts and breakfast cereals, have just enough salt to taunt your appetite center but not quite enough for you to notice it.

Fat, or oil, doesn't add taste directly, but it enhances the delivery of other tastes, so foods that don't really need to have sugar or added fat generally have both, delivering a tag-team blow to your hapless hypothalamus!

Whenever you see these taste triggers in places they really don't need to be, you are staring at the food industry's smoking gun: willful manipulation of the food supply to encourage, and even coerce, you to eat more than you should!

In the bloodstream: The stomach and intestines quickly convert the simple starch and sugar in the white bread into glucose, or blood sugar. The glucose seeps through the intestinal wall and into the bloodstream, sending blood sugar levels up. In response, the pancreas overproduces insulin, which moves glucose from the blood into muscles and other tissues. The insulin quickly drives down blood sugar, leading to more hunger.

On the other hand, the fiber in the oatmeal dissolves in water inside the intestines, where it creates a barrier through which nutrients must pass to get into the bloodstream, thus slowing the entrance of glucose into the blood. The result is a slower, lower rise in blood sugar; a slower release of insulin; no rapid surge and dip in blood sugar levels; and lasting fullness.

As you can see, what you eat has a powerful ability to influence how much you must eat to feel full and satisfied. You can't think yourself thin, as some books in the past have claimed. But by organizing the flavors in your foods, you *can* manipulate this complex series of chemicals and subdue the appetite center in your brain sooner, before you've overeaten.

THE EVOLUTION OF APPETITE

The secret behind the Flavor Point Diet is this simple fact: Our appetites are stimulated by flavor variety and lulled by flavor consistency. Why do we eat more when flavors are diverse? The answer to that question lies deep in human history and dates back to our hunting and gathering days.

The sweetness of chocolate, the saltiness of a pickle, the sourness of a lemon, and the bitterness of broccoli all affect the brain differently. Exactly how the human brain responds to these flavors is a product of millions of years of evolution. Our taste buds developed and evolved not to keep us happy but to keep us alive. They perform a vital function by assessing flavor, indicating what we should and shouldn't eat.

Over millions of years, our evolutionary biology has trained us to enjoy foods that keep us alive and abhor foods that don't. Most humans love sweet tastes, for example, and generally don't like bitter ones; one reason for this is that nature's poisons often come in bitter packages, while sweet foods are rarely if ever toxic.

We've also learned to delight in sweet tastes because sweet foods provided the calories our early ancestors needed to stay alive. The best source of fuel they could burn quickly to chase down an antelope or flee from a saber-toothed cat was sugar, found in nature in fruit and honey. The survival advantage of eating foods containing sugar has translated over the eons of natural selection into a strong preference for foods that taste sweet.

Much as we might think there is something intrinsically delicious

A Proclivity for Salt

Most of us prefer salty foods. In fact, without salt, food is often unpalatably bland. Why? Sodium was abundantly available in the oceans of our earliest origins and is thus a resource readily made use of in our physiology. A vital constituent of blood, sodium regulates the trans-membrane electrical potential that makes the nervous system work. This isn't because sodium is unique in its ability to perform these functions. Rather, it was an expedient choice as natural selection meandered haphazardly along, exploiting what was at hand.

When some distant cousin of ours grew tired of the incessant wet and decided land was the way to go, salt took on new significance. Because that expatriate from the briny deep didn't leave his or her metabolism in the sea, sodium remained a key constituent of animal physiology, even though it was suddenly and drastically less abundant. That, among other things, was the cost of drying out: Salt was essential but hard to find.

So we can thank our earliest land-dwelling ancestors for our proclivity for Doritos, pretzels, and pickles. We like salt. We seek salt. We always have.

Accounts from ancient Rome, for example, tell of nobles who were kidnapped and held for a ransom of salt and spices. The word *salary* comes from the Latin word for salt—*salarium*—because Roman soldiers were paid partly with this rare and precious commodity. Salzburg, Austria, may evoke scenes from *The Sound of Music,* but the name means "Salt City," attesting to a historically vital resource the region happens to provide.

about sugar, it's not really so. "Delicious" is simply how our brains interpret certain specific sensations our taste buds register as they interact with the chemical properties of food in our mouths. We learned to think of sugar as delicious because it helped our ancestors survive. Those of our ancestors who liked the tastes linked to survival—foods generally rich in sugar, salt, and/or fat and free of toxins—lived into adulthood and made babies. Those who didn't like such foods generally did neither.

Not only specific flavors but also a variety of flavors helped us survive. No one food houses all of the vitamins, minerals, and phytochemicals the human body needs to survive. Our early ancestors who got bored with berries—even if they were plentiful—and foraged for seeds and other foods consumed the variety of nutrients they needed to reproduce and pass on their genes to future generations. The early humans who ate berry after berry after berry—and nothing else—tended not to reproduce and pass on their genes. In this way, the traits and tendencies conducive to survival, favored by natural selection and encoded in our genes, have been passed down through the generations.

THE SCIENCE OF APPETITE

Sensory-specific satiety has been under study for decades; it's amazing, really, that hardly anyone has even heard of it! In fact, when I lecture to my fellow physicians and academic colleagues, I routinely ask who in the audience has heard of this critically important trait. If one hand out of hundreds ever goes up, it's generally someone who has heard me lecture before!

Yet sensory-specific satiety is nothing new. As I was writing this book, I searched the medical literature for every mention of every study done on the topic. I found hundreds. The earliest mention that I could find dates from 1981, the very early days of our current obesity epidemic. Articles on closely related topics date back even farther, to the mid-1970s.

I won't overwhelm you by listing all of the studies I found. I do, however, want to share four of the more compelling ones with you.

Satisfaction at the Flavor Point

THE FLAVOR FACTS

Name: Maureen McGowan

Age: 33

Hometown: Ansonia, Connecticut

Family status: Recently married

Occupation: Multiskilled technician

Starting weight: 209

Pounds lost: 17 in 12 weeks

Health stats: Energy level increased; waist measurement shrank 4½ inches

"I found out about Dr. Katz's program at the perfect time—6 months before my wedding.

"My problem was not overeating; I just used to eat all the wrong foods. Pizza, cheese steaks, hamburgers, and hot dogs were all regular staples of my diet.

"I was at my thinnest when I was in boot camp. Then, I only ate three meals a day and exercised constantly. When I got out of the military in 1995, I put on 40 pounds pretty fast.

"I tried many different programs in attempts to lose weight, but I always felt like I was starving. I'm not hungry at all on this program. It always seems like it's time to eat again—you have your breakfast, then a snack like fruit, then your lunch, then a snack like a fruit smoothie, and then it's time for dinner.

"A lot of times, I'm not even hungry for my nighttime snack. I

- In the mid-1980s, Barbara Rolls, PhD, then at Johns Hopkins University in Baltimore, and some colleagues gave 24 women a test meal of either soup or Jell-O. Some of the meals were high in calories, while others were low in calories. They all, however, tasted the same. An hour after the test meal, the researchers offered cheese and crackers to the study participants. They all ate roughly the same amount of cheese and crackers regardless of how many calories of soup or Jell-O they had eaten just an hour before. Why? Sensory-specific satiety! The cheese and don't feel like I'm depriving myself at all, and I see the pounds dropping off, which is motivating.

"On Dr. Katz's program, not only do I feel like I'm eating a lot, but I'm eating much better than I used to, and I really do enjoy these recipes. I enjoy the chicken dinners, and even though I'm not a fish eater, I really like the shrimp and tilapia dishes. And I *love* the pineapple shrimp.

"One of the best things about Dr. Katz's program is that I'm changing my overall eating habits. It's not a diet; it's a lifestyle change. Instead of butter, I'm using Smart Balance. Instead of vegetable oil, I'm using olive oil. I'm eating whole wheat pasta instead of regular pasta (and I don't even notice a difference!). I'm also eating a ton of vegetables—fresh asparagus, broccoli, cauliflower, you name it. And I know these are all things I'll be able to do continuously.

"People have definitely noticed my weight loss, particularly at work. Personally, I can see that my face and butt are thinner. Luckily, I carry my weight pretty evenly, so it's coming off all over my body. I just got into a pair of jeans I haven't been able to wear in 3 years!

"I still need to lose another 20 to 30 pounds, so I'm going to keep up with Dr. Katz's program. I love the results I've gotten so far, and I'm looking forward to seeing more." ▪

crackers provided a new taste, stimulating another appetite meter in the brain that had to register "full" before being turned off (see "Flavor Fluency" on page 5).

- In another interesting study completed around the same time, researchers fed 16 men and 16 women meals that varied in taste and texture. The participants found sweet foods less pleasurable when they had recently eaten sweet foods and salty foods less pleasurable when they had recently eaten salty foods.

- In 2001, researchers studied six lean and six overweight men on a metabolic ward. They varied the foods the men could eat each day and then let the participants eat as much as they wanted. The greater the variety of foods the researchers provided on any given day, the more total calories the men consumed and the greater their weight the next day! In fact, the men ate as much as 25 percent more calories when they had access to more foods. That's the equivalent of consuming 2,000 calories in a given day when you would normally eat only 1,600. Assuming you needed only 1,600 calories a day to maintain your weight, this type of daily excess would result in a gain of 36.5 pounds a year!
- Most recently, in 2004, researchers studied the effects of sensory-specific satiety in 21 overweight and 23 lean women. The investigators offered the women lunch, followed about 90 minutes later by a snack. The researchers varied the flavors and fat content of the foods for each meal and found that flavor had a far greater effect on appetite than fat content did. When the flavors in the lunch and snack were similar, the women ate less. When the flavors varied more between the lunch and snack, the women ate more!

As you can see, variety is indeed the spice of life—and our nutritional lives are becoming way too spicy! We now have access to a greater variety of foods and flavors every day than ever before in history. This flavor variety is a cause of obesity, including your personal weight-control struggles.

FROM PREHISTORIC TIMES TO A WORLD OF PLENTY

Originally, hunger was about survival. Hunger motivates us to eat because eating is essential. Sensations of fullness told our ancestors that they could stop risking their lives to find more food. Our brains evolved to deal with appetite in a world in which getting enough nutrients and calories was a constant challenge.

Today, that's no longer the case. Getting enough nutrients and calories is as easy as stopping at a takeout window. Yet, even though the modern world has changed, our brains have not. Our brains respond to this constant barrage of calories by telling us to eat more. Nothing in all of our historical experience has prepared us to resist food, because there has never, until now, been a reason to do so.

Here's what we're up against. In his excellent exposé, *Fast Food Nation*, investigative journalist Eric Schlosser describes in considerable detail how fast-food companies have engineered fast food to exploit every vulnerability of human taste and preference. These companies systematically test flavor additives with focus groups, tweaking foods until they become maximally pleasurable or, more bluntly, maximally addictive.

FLAVOR FLUENCY

HUNGER: The various sensations you feel when you confront a deficit in the fuel you need to keep yourself running.

This problem goes well beyond fast food. Along with my Yale colleague and friend, Kelly Brownell, PhD, I have long referred to the modern food environment as toxic.

The food industry bombards our taste buds with a staggering variety of flavors. These companies have processed sugar, salt, and harmful fats into foods that no longer bear any discernible resemblance to their origins. They've added flavor-enhancing chemicals. They've engineered salt into sweet foods, sugar into salty foods, and an intoxicating combination of flavors into the contents of every bag, box, meal, and snack.

From potato chips and french fries to cookies and ice cream, many foods have become arguably as addictive—and, in the long run, nearly as bad for you—as cigarettes. This type of processing raises the Flavor Point. With so much flavor variety, it's almost impossible not to overeat.

Is this intentional? Probably. The connection between flavor variety and overeating has appeared in medical studies for more than 20 years.

How Flavors Affect Eating

Many years ago, scientists identified only four major taste categories: sweet, sour, salty, and bitter. Now, science tells us there are at least six distinct taste categories, the two additions being savory (also called umami) and astringent. Perhaps someday, we'll know of even more. Our ability to appreciate the many subtle variations in the flavors of foods results from our perception of these categories of taste, combined with our interpretation of aromas. Smell contributes a lot to our sense of taste, which is why eating with a stuffy nose tends to be so unsatisfying.

Although sensory-specific satiety drives us to prefer a variety of tastes, not all tastes are created equal. Sweet stimulates our appetites the most. This makes perfect sense. Breast milk is sweet. In nature, sweet foods are scarce and include excellent sources of quick energy, such as ripe fruits and wild honey. Few toxic substances in nature taste sweet, so there are many good reasons for us to be born with a sweet tooth (or gums, as the case may be!).

Salt also stimulates appetite. Although humans aren't born with a predilection for salty food, we readily acquire it. The same appears to be true for the savory quality of protein sources such as meat and cheese. In contrast, bitter and astringent tastes tend to suppress appetite, at least until we acquire a preference for them. For example, coffee and beer are acquired tastes for many people, but once we learn to like them, we may like them quite a lot!

Have the smart and well-paid nutritional biochemists working for the food industry failed to appreciate its significance? That would be hard for me to believe.

Is the modern food industry actually involved in some kind of conspiracy? Do executives meet in boardrooms and exchange dark secrets about how to addict the country's population to their foods? No one knows, but it would require a good deal of vacuous inattention on the part of a food company executive not to appreciate the potential utility of sensory-specific satiety in the effective peddling of an excess of wares. Because vacuous inattention is not a trait common among successful business executives, I'm guessing that the food industry quickly figured out what sensory-specific satiety could mean to their bottom line.

An investigative journalist—perhaps Eric Schlosser, if he's inclined to write the sequel to *Fast Food Nation*—might find what I don't have the time, skills, or inclination to look for: long-hidden documents lurking in a drawer at some large food or restaurant company that signify the willful processing of hidden flavors into foods to stimulate overconsumption.

I don't need these documents to know that the practice is widespread. I just need the nutrition facts and ingredient labels that the FDA requires on packaged foods. I can see right there that processing has crossed over to the dark side. When breakfast cereals are salty, and savory snacks provide sugar in doses suitable for dessert, I can see the smoke from the gun, whether or not I can find the bullet or have the evidence needed to indict the shooter.

Take monosodium glutamate, for example. This ingredient does more than make foods taste salty. Glutamate, an amino acid, is responsible for a unique flavor category all its own, known as umami, which signifies the kind of savory flavor we taste in cheese and meat. It's hard to define, but you know it when you taste it! Because most people like it, it's being processed into ever more foods.

Some of these flavors aren't really intended to be tasted at all! Some so-called flavor enhancers are hidden. They stimulate additional appetite meters in our brains, and stimulate us to eat more, but we don't actually taste them.

For example, many breakfast cereals taste sweet, but they actually contain quite a bit of salt, almost as much as potato chips or pretzels. Even though you don't notice a salty flavor (after all, who wants a breakfast cereal to taste salty?), it doesn't escape your appetite center. We taste the sugar in breakfast cereal, and that activates one appetite meter. Although the sweetness of sugar masks the saltiness of the salt, the salt activates another appetite meter. The activation of two distinct appetite meters by two distinct flavors adds up to a bigger appetite. You'll consume more cereal before both of the meters register fullness.

Just about every single shrink-wrapped, boxed, or bagged food you find on supermarket shelves contains this enticing sugar-salt combination. Foods that taste sweet contain salt. Foods that taste salty contain sugar. Most of these foods also contain an array of artificial flavors. Added to-

A Short History of Food Processing

Even in prehistory, food was processed. Humans may have frozen and smoke-cured their food as far back as the last Ice Age. They at times ground wild plants into flour, cooked meat, and smoked and dried foods to preserve them. All of this was a departure from eating totally unprocessed food as it was found.

Processing throughout most of history was about making enough food available to forestall genuine hunger. It was about preventing spoilage. It was about making food safer.

That changed in the latter half of the 20th century. The United States now produces, after accounting for export, roughly 3,800 calories each day for every man, woman, and child in the country. Other than for the few of you who play for the NFL, run ultramarathons, or routinely trek in the Himalayas, this calorie load grossly exceeds the needs of most people. In response, the primary incentive for the processing of food changed from making enough food safely available to making unsafe amounts of food all but irresistible.

Flavor Pointer

GETTING ADDICTED TO HEALTH

Even the most powerful habit-forming substances do their damage only when you use them frequently and at fairly high doses. In this way, the need for the substance goes up and up and up. As need rises, however, satisfaction falls.

The same is true of flavors. Most of us have so much sugar and salt in our diets that we don't even notice them in moderate amounts; we taste them only when the dose is quite high. As a result, we need more and more and more added sugar and salt to reach our flavor thresholds, the point at which we feel satisfied with these flavors. Eating ever-higher doses of sugar and salt simply propagates their addictive influence, making us turn to less wholesome, more processed, higher-calorie foods.

Here's the good news: Health can be just as habit forming! The Flavor Point Diet leads you steadily to foods that are less processed and have less added sugar, salt, and harmful fats. As you acclimate to these lower flavor thresholds, not only will you completely recover from your flavor addictions, you will also find that it takes less and less and less of these ingredients to satisfy you. You will start to find that the sweets you used to enjoy now taste too sweet and the salty snacks too salty. As you choose and acclimate to more wholesome foods, you will rehabilitate your taste buds! You don't need to give up the foods you prefer. You will instead come to prefer the more wholesome foods that now, along with better health, are your new habit! Once this habit is formed, you won't need to follow the flavor themes consciously—you'll begin to choose Flavor Point–friendly foods automatically, for life.

gether, this flavor excess stimulates a number of appetite meters in the brain, all of which must register fullness before you feel satisfied. Under these conditions, no amount of willpower will hold you to a small serving of potato chips or cheese puffs.

OVERCOMING MODERN TEMPTATIONS

I have long used the image of polar bears in the Sahara to help my patients understand why weight control is so difficult and frustrating. So let's consider polar bears for a moment. These marvels of survival flourish in one of Earth's harshest climates. They are made for the cold. They have double-layer coats, insulating inner hairs, and hollow outer hairs that funnel solar radiation to their skin. Their black skin absorbs all wavelengths of sunlight. Polar bears soak up and retain heat with extraordinary efficiency.

Imagine what would happen if polar bears suddenly found themselves in the Sahara on a summer day. In a world of abundant heat, they would quickly find that the tendency to absorb and retain heat would be their undoing. They would overheat, not for lack of willpower or because of greed, gluttony, or laziness. No, they would soak up heat because that's what polar bears do.

People overeat for all the same reasons that polar bears overheat. Just as polar bears conserve heat, our ancestors conserved food energy. Polar bears have physiologies designed to thrive when available heat is limited; they soak up and conserve warmth. Humans have physiologies designed to thrive when calories are scarce; we soak up and conserve calories, running quite well on relatively few and storing the rest as body fat to use when needed. Just as polar bears are undone by their ability to store heat when heat is suddenly abundant, humans don't cope well when food is suddenly available in excess. We tend to overeat!

One of two solutions can fix the mismatch between human metabolism and the modern environment. The first and most fundamental is to restore the environment to its former state. Many of my most esteemed colleagues are completely devoted to this cause, working to change food industry practices, urban planning, and government policy (see, for example, *Food Fight* by Dr. Brownell and *Food Politics* by New York University professor Marion Nestle, PhD).

Despite the best efforts of some of the best people in science and public health, I have this advice for you: Don't hold your breath!

Changing the world is neither quick nor easy, and sometimes it may be nearly impossible. It seems rather unlikely, for example, that we humans will ever abandon time- and laborsaving devices, such as snowblowers and e-mail, that contribute to our obesity.

So that leaves us with the other way: adapting to live successfully in our new environment. Most diets do not empower you to outthink the forces and sources of weight gain. Most diets are short-term solutions to a profound and permanent problem. Think of yourself as a polar bear in the Sahara and the typical diet as a big block of ice. You're given the ice and invited to climb on. It's cool, comfortable, and instantly rewarding.

But what happens to a block of ice under the relentless Sahara sun? It melts. You haven't really fallen off the diets you've tried before; instead, they've disappeared out from under you, never offering anything meaningful and permanent in the first place.

The Flavor Point Diet is not a block of ice. Rather, it provides an exit strategy from the desert heat. Using the power of your brain, the Flavor Point Diet lets you turn the very forces that conspired to produce epidemic obesity—and your own struggle with weight—to your advantage.

WHY WILLPOWER DOESN'T WORK

I'm willing to bet that you have plenty of willpower. You probably have at least the average endowment of discipline and motivation. You're not lazy. You are not the problem. The problem lies in the foods that surround—and tempt—you day in and day out. As you now understand, however, you need more than willpower to overcome the addictiveness of the modern food supply. You need flavor organization.

In this modern environment, there are powerful forces working against your best efforts at weight control. You can't just make up your mind to overcome this genetic wiring. Willpower might work for a day or a week or even a month. Over time, however, your genetics will overpower your willpower, causing you to backslide.

That's where the Flavor Point Diet comes in. You can eat less but feel just as full and satisfied. Indeed, there's only one way to overcome evolutionary biology: You must eat in a way that triggers that appetite center in your brain to tell the rest of your body that you're satisfied with less. To eat less, you need more than your willpower and determination on your side. You need your brain.

The Flavor Point Meal Plan teaches you to choose foods free of superfluous flavor enhancers, foods that don't overstimulate your appetite center and lead to excessive eating. It teaches you how to choose foods based on flavor themes that tame your appetite and then transition off of those themes to a basic pattern of foods and flavors you can sustain forever. By focusing on organizing the flavors in your diet, you wind up improving everything about the foods you buy, stock, prepare, and order. More important, you can follow the Flavor Point Diet for life.

That's the power of neuroscience. That's the power of using the hardwiring of your brain, rather than just making up your mind, to lose weight and keep it off. That's the power of lowering your Flavor Point. Let's turn to Chapter 2 to learn more about how you can use your brain to turn down your appetite.

OTHER APPETITE TRIGGERS

Although many variables influence how much you eat, flavor matters most.

Because my wife, Catherine, is French, our family meals all begin with a hearty *"Bon appétit,"* which means "Good appetite." As you've learned, however, not everything about appetite is good! A great many pressures cause our appetites to behave badly.

Among those pressures, flavor variety ranks as the most important, but I'd be oversimplifying things if I told you it was the only one. Social, environmental, psychological, economic, and biological factors all influence how much humans eat—and overeat. In addition to flavor, the volume of a food, the number of calories it contains, and its nutrient content all influence the Flavor Point. The good news: When you organize the flavors in your diet, all of these other appetite-stimulating variables fall into place! Let's take a closer look.

THE VOLUME CONNECTION

The volume of a food refers to how much space a fairly typical serving of the food takes up. A low-volume food would be something like cheese, which packs lots of calories into a small space. A high-volume food would be lettuce, which takes up lots of space but provides very few calories. High-volume foods are generally also referred to as energy dilute, meaning that they have relatively few calories for any given unit of volume; low-volume foods tend to be energy dense. Volume can be altered by adding water, so, for example, chicken soup is a higher-volume and less energy-dense food than chicken.

I mentioned the stomach hormone ghrelin in Chapter 1. Levels of this appetite-stimulating hormone remain high until food stretches the wall of your stomach, making you feel full. This stretch reflex helps explain why Barbara Rolls, PhD, and her colleagues at Pennsylvania State University in University Park have linked high-volume, low-calorie foods with reduced appetite and increased satiety. These foods take up a lot of room in your stomach, triggering the stretch reflex in the stomach wall long before you've overeaten. On the other hand, the same researchers have found that low-volume, high-calorie foods, such as potato chips and french fries, encourage overeating, probably because you must eat a lot more of them to trigger the same reflex.

In one study published in 2003, Dr. Rolls and her colleagues offered various types of soup to 36 women over several days. When the researchers doubled the volume of the soup but kept calories constant, the women felt full faster and stopped eating after consuming fewer calories. When the researchers doubled the calories in the soup but kept the volume the same, the women consumed more calories.

In a related study, the researchers offered 20 men a milk-based drink, followed by lunch and then dinner. When the drink was relatively low in volume, the men ate more for lunch and dinner that day, consuming more calories than usual. When the men had shakes that were higher in volume but had the same number of calories, they ate less at the subsequent meals.

In yet another study, with 28 men, the investigators varied the volume of a yogurt drink by putting air into it, keeping everything else constant. Even when they changed only the air content, the higher-volume drink caused the subjects to eat less during that day!

These and other studies clearly demonstrate the powerful effect that food volume has on appetite. This important concept is the basis for Dr. Rolls's excellent book *The Volumetrics Weight-Control Plan: Feel Full on Fewer Calories.*

High-volume foods can certainly help you in your quest to fill up on fewer calories, but is volume more important than flavor? I don't think so. If I did, I wouldn't have written this book. By controlling the variety of flavors in your meals and snacks, you avoid stimulating multiple appetite meters at any one time (see "Flavor Fluency"). Then, by incorporating high-volume foods into your diet, you satisfy the meters that are turned on with fewer calories. By activating fewer meters and turning off your activated meters sooner, you will create a shortcut to the Flavor Point.

Luckily, you don't need to earn a degree in biochemistry to use volume to your advantage. Foods with simple, wholesome ingredients and simple flavors tend to be high in volume. You can trick your brain (and stomach) by adding water and air to certain foods, increasing volume without adding calories. So make your soups soupier and your smoothies bubblier!

FLAVOR FLUENCY

APPETITE: A desire for a particular food or a craving for a particular taste. Many circumstances influence appetite, including exposure to certain foods, timing of the meal or snack, and tradition or convention. The familiarity of food, its palatability (which incorporates taste and texture, appearance and aroma), its convenience and cost, and its place in our culture also influence appetite. Of all of these variables, flavor exerts the strongest influence on appetite.

THE CALORIE CONNECTION

We tend to eat more than we should when the foods we choose are energy dense, meaning that they pack a lot of calories into a relatively small serving.

To understand why, imagine for a moment that it's 3:00 p.m. You're

(continued on page 29)

Satisfaction at the Flavor Point

> **THE FLAVOR FACTS**
>
> Name: Nancy Schebell
>
> Age: 36
>
> Hometown: Naugatuck, Connecticut
>
> Family status: Divorced with three children, ages 3, 7, and 11
>
> Occupation: X-ray technician
>
> Starting weight: 238
>
> Pounds lost: 16 in 12 weeks
>
> Health stats: Blood pressure dropped 5 points; waist measurement shrank 7 inches; 4 percent decline in body fat

"The last time I was thin, I was a senior in high school. After having three kids and going to numerous ball games and eating junk regularly over the years, the weight just came on. I had tried Atkins in the past and I was a freak on it; after 2 weeks without carbs, I was miserable and I gave up.

"Dr. Katz told us in the begin-ning that this is a way of life and not a diet. He was right. I really love this program, and I think it's something I'll be able to stick with for life.

"I now love grocery shopping. When I go, I spend a lot of time browsing, and I'm always looking for something different to try in the health food section. I *want* to find new foods that are good for me.

"Not only are the recipes really tasty, they're doable for a family. My kids are ages 3, 7, and 11 and they love the foods, especially the fish. We had never eaten tuna before, but when I made it for the plan, my kids loved it. They also love the oat bran pretzels as a snack (as do I).

"As far as the ease of the meals, I was never big on cooking, and these recipes are pretty simple for me. My mom is impressed that I'm cooking! Overall, I think my favorite flavor themes were the vegetable ones—the tomato and mushroom.

"For breakfast, I make an omelet or a smoothie and take it to work. For lunch, I usually choose one of the flavor-friendly options and have a salad with grilled chicken or tuna. I sometimes eat the hummus sandwiches for lunch. Then I make the recipes specified on the meal plan for dinner.

"I used to crave chocolate a lot. Since I started the program, my cravings have stopped. Instead of sweets, I now opt for a cracker with some hummus on it or a handful of Kashi TLC crackers, carrots, or grape tomatoes. I always drink green tea because Dr. Katz told us it helps make you feel full, and it really works.

"Dr. Katz taught me to honor the flavor that I crave. He says if you want something salty, eat something salty, but don't eat something sweet right after it. The same thing goes for craving sweets—just eat something sweet without following it up with something salty. Otherwise, you won't be satisfied. He's right. It works.

"I also drink a lot of water now. I used to drink a lot of soda. I would always drink my eight glasses of water, but I'd drink soda at lunch and dinner. Not anymore. Even at lunch, I drink water. I find the soda too sweet.

"I am amazed at how full I am. I didn't make the desserts because most of the time, I was satisfied with dinner. I didn't need anything else.

"I feel so much better on this program; I have much more energy, and I've been walking between 2 and 4 miles every day. My clothes fit better, and people have been saying, 'Oh, my God—look at you! You're so much thinner. You look so good.' My coworkers have been particularly supportive. And a lot of people have asked me about the program that I'm on; they can't wait to try it, too!"

The Universe of Foods

Try to choose foods from group B in the chart below. For overall health, the next best group is group A, foods dense in both nutrients and calories. Foods low in both nutrients and calories (group D) may not foster weight gain directly but can do so indirectly, as in the case of diet soda (see "Why Sugar Substitutes Don't Work" on page 34). These foods and beverages also offer few if any health benefits. Then there's group C: foods high in calories and low in nutrients. These badlands of the food universe are home to just about every junk food you can think of. If you spend too much time in group C, you'll fire up your brain's appetite meters, moving you away from the Flavor Point.

	HIGH NUTRIENT DENSITY	LOW NUTRIENT DENSITY
HIGH ENERGY DENSITY	A. High in both nutrients and calories: nuts, seeds, olives, avocados, and some animal foods, such as fatty fish	C. Low in nutrients, high in calories: fast food, fried foods, chips, deli meats, soda, most candies, doughnuts, muffins, cookies, crackers, cream sauces, butter, mayonnaise, etc.
LOW ENERGY DENSITY	B. High in nutrients, low in calories: vegetables, fruits, and whole grains	D. Low in both nutrients and calories: diet soda and other diet beverages; celery; iceberg lettuce; fat-free, reduced-calorie spreads and dressings; etc.

ready to take a break and are in the mood for a snack. You have a simple choice: an apple or a slice of Cheddar cheese. Both provide 100 calories, but you'll swallow the cheese in a bite or two, whereas the apple will take you a while to eat. What do you think will happen if you opt for the cheese? Will you stop at just one slice? Probably not.

When foods pack lots of calories in a small space, as cheese does, it's easy to overeat. Because an apple takes longer to eat, your brain has time to register fullness. The apple's fiber and water also stimulate stretch receptors in the stomach more quickly.

Because fat has 9 calories per gram compared with carbohydrate or protein's 4 calories per gram, foods high in fat are energy dense. Processed foods with lots of sugar come in a close second. Processed foods loaded with both fat and sugar have dense concentrations of calories that are especially palatable and hard to resist. Because fiber takes up space in food but provides no calories, simply increasing your fiber consumption could help turn down your appetite—yet our highly processed food supply does just the opposite. Processed foods have been stripped of their fiber!

The overprocessing and increasing energy density of the American diet is one of the leading causes of epidemic obesity. Energy-dense foods make it easy to squeeze too many calories into your stomach within a small amount of time and space. There is very little obesity seen in societies that rely on energy-dilute foods. Regrettably, there are fewer and fewer such societies as both highly processed, energy-dense foods and obesity relentlessly take over our planet!

The Flavor Point Diet relies on foods that are naturally low in fat, such as fruits, vegetables, and whole grains. While reducing the amount of fat you consume can also reduce the energy density of your diet, it works only if you consume naturally low-fat foods. Too often, dieters turn to processed low-fat and fat-free foods (think of Snackwells). Because these foods contain lots of sugar, they are often nearly as energy dense as their high-fat cousins! Another consideration is that cutting out too much fat makes eating less enjoyable and renders a diet unsustainable. The Flavor Point Diet avoids this mistake.

(continued on page 32)

What Makes You Eat

Although the Flavor Point Meal Plan addresses all of the following influences on appetite to give you maximum control and mastery over your Flavor Point, you need to focus on only one thing: flavor. When you choose simply flavored foods, all of the other influences fall into place.

INFLUENCE	HOW TO USE IT
Sensory-specific satiety	Avoid excess flavor variety in meals, snacks, and processed into individual foods; group flavors into themes (see Chapter 3 for more details).
Energy density	Foods that pack lots of calories into small spaces are less filling and satisfying than foods that distribute calories in larger volumes. Avoid or limit highly processed foods that have lots of calories from fat and sugar and are devoid of water and fiber.
Volume	Foods high in volume, such as vegetables, fruits, soups, and stews, fill you up with fewer calories. These wholesome foods are also generally rich in nutrients. Make them a regular part of a healthful diet.
Protein	Calorie for calorie, protein is the most filling of the nutrient categories, but too much can be harmful. The Flavor Point Meal Plan delivers protein at the upper end of the range recommended for lasting good health.

INFLUENCE	HOW TO USE IT
Glycemic load	A better measure than the glycemic index, the glycemic load indicates how much foods tend to raise blood sugar. Swings in blood sugar over-stimulate appetite and contribute to weight gain. The Flavor Point Meal Plan emphasizes foods with a low glycemic load. By choosing less processed foods, you will lower the glycemic load of your diet, speeding you to the Flavor Point.
Fiber content	Fiber reduces your risk of heart disease, diabetes, and cancer as well as helping to control appetite. Most people, however, eat less than half the recommended amount of about 30 milligrams a day. The Flavor Point Meal Plan consistently delivers an ideal dose of fiber each day. Found in cereal grains, fruit, vegetables, nuts, seeds, beans, and lentils, fiber is plentiful in the Flavor Point Diet.
Fat content	Fat is less filling, calorie for calorie, than either protein or carbohydrate. It's also more energy dense, packing more calories into a smaller volume. Fat also serves as a vehicle for flavors. Sweet foods taste even sweeter, for example, when they are made with oil. The oil distributes the sweetness throughout the mouth. Even though added oils may not add a specific flavor to food, they enhance the potency of other added flavors. For these reasons, the Flavor Point Diet emphasizes foods naturally low in fat. The fats in this diet are almost all of the healthful, unsaturated variety.

THE MACRONUTRIENT CONNECTION

The appetite meters in our brains respond somewhat differently to the different nutrient classes we consume. For example, the more protein we eat, the more readily the meters register "Full." Although no one knows precisely why, I can guess. We need protein every day for good health, and our ancestors had to hunt—a dangerous activity—to procure it. So it makes sense that our brains and appetites not only motivate us to seek out protein but also let us know when we've had enough. Risking life and limb for protein we didn't need would be almost as ill advised as not risking life and limb for it at all.

Whatever the reasons, the science is clear that calorie for calorie, protein is the most satiating (filling) of the nutrient classes, followed by complex carbohydrates (those rich in fiber, such as whole grains, vegetables, and fruits), then simple carbohydrates (white flour and products containing added sugar), and finally, fat. This means it takes more calories from fat than from either carbohydrate or protein to make us feel comparably full. Because fat is the least satiating of the nutrient classes, high-fat foods can easily make you eat more than you intend to.

That said, when foods are mixed together, as they always are in any reasonable diet, even the satiating power of protein is reduced. Thus, relying on a low-carbohydrate, high-protein diet for weight control is not likely to work very well, and such diets are generally unbalanced. Finally, because restrictive diets get tedious, they tend to backfire. You lose weight for as long as you can stand the tedium, but when you can stand it no longer and go off the diet, you gain back the weight with interest.

The Flavor Point Diet avoids these pitfalls, providing the perfect balance of macronutrients for nutrition and health while controlling appetite with the powerful and permanent force of flavor. The breakdown, designed for lifelong health and weight control, looks like this.

- Roughly 55 percent of calories from mostly complex carbohydrate
- Roughly 20 percent of calories from lean sources of protein

Flavor Pointer

A RECKONING OF RENEGADE CALORIES

On the Flavor Point Diet, you needn't count calories, because you'll use food to fill up on fewer calories automatically. That said, you do need to stay vigilant. Don't let hidden, overlooked calories sneak into your day and onto your hips or waist. Pay attention to handfuls of nuts or chips or candies you may tend to grab on the go. Be attentive to spreads, dressings, and sauces. And don't forget the calories you're drinking! Counting calories for weight control? Tiresome. You can fuhgeddaboudit, as long as you remember that all calories do count!

- Roughly 25 percent of calories from fat, most from healthful sources such as vegetable oils, nuts, seeds, and fish and very little from animal sources or processed foods

Here's my reasoning. First, this is the dietary pattern that many major health organizations and an abundance of research indicate is optimal for lifelong health. Second, foods high in complex carbohydrates, such as vegetables, fruits, and whole grains, tend to be rich in fiber, water, or both. Fiber may be particularly important because it increases food volume without added calories and can slow the absorption of nutrients into the bloodstream, thereby lowering blood sugar and stabilizing blood insulin levels. For lasting weight control, it makes far more sense to choose carbohydrate foods wisely than to simply abandon them altogether.

There's one caveat to all of this. High-carbohydrate foods are more filling and satiating than high-fat foods only if they contain water and fiber. Once processing removes the natural water and fiber content of a high-carbohydrate food and then adds sugar and refined starch, these foods trigger overeating just as fatty foods do. In other words, those reduced-fat Oreos aren't doing your waistline any good!

Why Sugar Substitutes Don't Work

Although sugar and fat substitutes allow you to enjoy sweet and creamy tastes and textures without consuming sweet and creamy calories, the use of these substitutes often backfires.

Studies show that we often compensate for these missing calories by eating more at other times. A fascinating study on this matter was recently carried out with mice. Researchers fed genetically identical mice either diet soda or regular soda and then offered the rodents sweet gruel. The mice given the diet soda overate the gruel and became obese, whereas the mice given the regular soda were better able to judge the calories in the gruel, ate less of it, and stayed lean! The artificial sweetener in the diet soda disrupted the mice's ability to regulate their intake of calories.

All artificial sweeteners can produce this effect. The more you eat of any desired flavor over time, the higher it tends to drive your threshold for satisfaction. Although the science of sensory-specific satiety proves that eating the same flavor in one sitting turns down the appetite, eating a lot of the same flavor on a regular basis raises your appetite for that flavor. In the case of artificial sweeteners, this propagates a sweet tooth. The best way to tame a sweet tooth is not by feeding it but by weaning it. The Flavor Point Diet will help you remove sugar from places in your diet it simply doesn't need to be, such as in breads, sauces, spreads, and dressings. As long as you don't replace this sweet taste with artificial sweeteners, you'll reduce your exposure not only to sugar but also to sweetness. That lowers your preference for sweet tastes so you're satisfied with less.

THE GLYCEMIC CONNECTION

The glycemic index is a measure of how much various foods raise blood sugar levels in comparison to a specific food used as a reference standard (usually a slice of white bread). In general, foods with high glycemic indexes are considered bad for weight control because a rapid rise in blood sugar leads to a brisk rise in blood insulin, which in turn may increase appetite by causing blood sugar levels to dip back down. In contrast, foods with low glycemic indexes are generally considered to help you lose weight because they produce smaller, slower variations in blood sugar and insulin levels. Although some studies show that foods with high glycemic indexes tend to be less filling than foods with low glycemic indexes, you really can't use the index to guide your food choices—for several reasons.

Perhaps the most straightforward reason is that the glycemic index compares a fixed dose of sugar in one food with the same dose in another. This is unfair! Getting the test dose of sugar from ice cream requires eating very little ice cream, whereas getting it from carrots requires eating a whole lot of carrots. The result? Ice cream has a lower glycemic index than white bread, and carrots have a higher one!

Unless you're prepared to believe that eating lots of ice cream and steering clear of carrots will enhance your health or control your weight, I trust you can see the limitations of the glycemic index. Still, the effects of foods on blood sugar and blood insulin levels are important and can play a role in weight loss. As I mentioned in Chapter 1, to turn down appetite, you need slow, even increases in blood sugar and insulin.

A more useful measure for guiding dietary choices is something called the glycemic load, which takes into account the dose of sugar found naturally in a food. The glycemic index compares sugar in foods the same way a tape measure compares the heights of a boy and a man. Let's say a 35-year-old man is 5 feet 2 inches tall, and a 5-year-old boy is 4 feet 6 inches tall. The tape measure tells us the man is tall and the boy short. In fact, the opposite is true! For his age, the man is relatively short; for his age, the boy is quite tall. Adjusting height for age reveals the truth about

Satisfaction at the Flavor Point

THE FLAVOR FACTS

Name: Chris Cornell

Age: 25

Hometown: West Haven, Connecticut

Family status: Married

Occupation: Field service technician

Starting weight: 217

Pounds lost: 10 in 12 weeks

Health stats: Blood pressure dropped 7 points; resting heart rate improved; $5\frac{1}{2}$ percent decline in body fat

---

"I was looking for something new—something that would not just help me lose weight but make me feel better overall. I had tried losing weight on my own and had also tried Dr. Phil's program with modest success, but I didn't stick with it. When I heard about Dr. Katz's plan, I decided to give it a try. I'm really glad I did, because it works.

"Overall, my favorite thing about the program is the food. It's great, especially the fish dishes. And most of the recipes are fast and pretty easy to make. I often try to prepare some of the dishes ahead of time, so they're ready to go when I need them, which makes things even simpler.

"For breakfast and lunch, I use the Flavor-Friendly Alternatives, cereal and fruit in the morning and a salad for lunch. For dinners, the seafood dishes are my favorites, especially the almond tilapia and the grilled shrimp. When I need a snack, I usually reach for raw veggies, fruit, or yogurt.

"I have also discovered new foods I never would have thought taste good. Alexia french fries have become a staple of my diet, and I found that Newman's Own light salad dressing is actually quite good!

"A number of people have commented on my weight loss and told me I look smaller, which has reinforced that the program is working. My clothes also fit much better. Plus, I have more energy now, which is a bonus.

"In a perfect world, I'd like to be 180, but I'm happy with the amount of weight I've lost in 12 weeks with Dr. Katz's program." ■

height much more accurately. The glycemic load does the same for the effects of food on blood sugar and insulin responses; it adjusts the effects of the food according to how its sugar content is concentrated. Whereas the glycemic index of carrots is comparable to that of soda, the glycemic load of carrots is less than one-tenth as much! Now that makes sense.

To use glycemic load to your advantage, you don't have to take a glycemic load chart with you each time you head to the supermarket. To consume a diet low in foods with high glycemic loads, you need only limit highly processed foods and maximize your consumption of vegetables, fruits, whole grains, and lean protein. The Flavor Point Diet does exactly that!

THE POWER OF FLAVOR, PLUS MORE

The Flavor Point Diet meal plan uses all of these important appetite regulators—volume, energy density, macronutrient content, glycemic load, and more—to help you fill up on the fewest calories. Of all the variables that influence appetite, however, flavor exerts the strongest influence, both in those of us who struggle with our weight and in those of us who do not. More important, foods with simple, satisfying flavors tend to include all of the appetite-subduing variables I just mentioned. In other words, when you follow the Flavor Point Meal Plan and subscribe to the Flavor Point principles, you will soon learn that you don't need to pay attention to calories, volume, macronutrients, and other variables. Appetite management will happen naturally, behind the scenes, without effort on your part.

Quite simply, flavor is the most important aspect of food. By using flavor strategically, you can use your meals to turn off your appetite center sooner. Turn to Chapter 3 to find out how.

Satisfaction at the Flavor Point

THE FLAVOR FACTS

Name: Brenda Gibbs

Age: 57

Hometown: Woodbridge, Connecticut

Family status: Married with two children, ages 18 and 28

Occupation: Registered nurse

Starting weight: 334

Pounds lost: 17 in 12 weeks

Health stats: Blood pressure dropped 28 points; resting heart rate decreased; blood sugar levels improved; waist measurement shrank $4\frac{1}{2}$ inches

"I was in a car accident about 6 years ago, and a resulting back injury made movement difficult. The less I moved, the more weight I put on, and the more weight I put on, the less I moved. It was a vicious cycle.

"Before I started the program, I ate anything and everything I wanted—cheeseburgers, fries, pasta salad, you name it. I would also keep a few Oreos next to my bed, and if I woke up hungry, I would eat them and go back to sleep.

"As a result, I put on *a lot* of weight since the accident, and I finally said to myself, 'Something is going to have to change, or you're going to die.' I have a 7-year-old granddaughter and a son who's going to college. I wanted to be around for them. So when Dr. Katz's program came along, I decided to give it a try. I reasoned with myself, 'If I can change what I put in my mouth, maybe I will feel physically better and want to move more.' That's exactly what this program has done for me.

"Now that I'm into it, this new eating plan has become a habit, and I love it. I really do. My husband does the cooking, so he had to stock the kitchen with these new ingredients over the first 2 weeks, but once he did that, he found the recipes to be pretty easy. He hasn't stuck to the program religiously, but he eats some of the dishes and finds them flavorful.

"The foods on the program please all your senses—sight, smell, and taste. And I don't feel like I'm on a strict regimen. This weekend, I went to a cookout, and instead of having a hamburger on a bun, I just had a small burger without the bun and a salad.

"And there is so *much* food that I can't eat it all. For breakfast, I usually eat cereal, but I occasionally make one of the more elaborate recipes, like the French toast made with the whole grain bread or the whole wheat waffles. I don't miss the bagel with butter and jelly I used to have for breakfast. The lentil salads are great for lunch, as are the egg and tuna salads. Because I'm heading to bed around lunchtime (I work third shift), I usually eat a few of the Wasa crackers with hummus and sprouts and I'm fine.

"My favorite dinners are the Pasta Fagioli with Spinach Marinara Sauce and the Portobello Mushrooms with Walnut Stuffing. I could eat the portobello dish 24/7. It's wonderful. To me, it tastes like stuffed lobster.

"I've also discovered some great new products, like the Alexia fries and the California veggie burgers; they are to die for. I bought Boca ground soy burgers, and my husband mixed them with vegetables and bulgur wheat, and it was like an American chop suey—out of sight! I didn't know I wasn't eating meat. And I love the Kashi cereal and the bulgur wheat. There are a lot of foods on this program that I never thought I'd eat, but I love them.

"One of the best things about Dr. Katz's program is how I look. I've gotten so many compliments. People say, 'Brenda, you look wonderful. You look so healthy.' My mother has been inspired to try it, too. She started 3 weeks ago and has lost 11 pounds so far!

"Physically, I feel great. I sleep better, and my energy level is incredible. At work, I used to delegate a lot of duties to other people, but now, I just get up and do a lot of the things myself.

"Both my husband and I are amazed that I not only stuck to the program for the first 12 weeks but also want to continue with it. My husband recently said, 'Brenda, I'm really shocked and pleased to see that you've taken to this so easily and that you're enjoying it. I'm a wholehearted advocate of this program!'"

REACHING THE FLAVOR POINT

Fill up on fewer calories in three easy steps.

Now that you have a working knowledge of the neuroscience of appetite and of the food industry's exploitation of your metabolic vulnerabilities, you may understand why weight control has been so difficult and elusive. That's the bad news.

Here's the good news: You can take advantage of the science of sensory-specific satiety and turn down your appetite without losing out on the flavor of your meals. You don't have to give up your favorite foods. In fact, quite to the contrary, you're going to eat more of them. You don't need to spend more time in the kitchen or at the supermarket. You needn't refrain from eating out. You don't have to prepare one meal for yourself and another for your family. You can subdue your appetite center with easy to prepare, tasty foods that even your children will love!

The Flavor Point Meal Plan is completely balanced, totally satisfying, absolutely healthful, permanently sustainable, and wonderfully effective for weight loss and lasting weight control. The plan helps turn down appetite on two levels.

1. You learn to drape a flavor theme over your meals, cooking simply but deliciously flavored foods that help trigger fullness with fewer calories.

Soup, Salad, Sandwich: At, or Beside, the Point?

As Shakespeare once asked, "What's in a name?" Potentially, a great deal of deception. Some foods, such as salad, sound weight-loss friendly, but not all are. The same goes for soup and sandwiches. Take a look at this chart to see which ingredients form the soup, salad, and sandwich categories that help you lower your Flavor Point and which do not. It's not what you call your food but what's in it that counts! Choose wisely.

FOOD	AT THE FLAVOR POINT	BESIDE THE POINT
SOUP	Vegetable or defatted chicken stock, clear broth, or tomato puree as a base; abundance of fresh vegetables and natural spices to taste	Cream, beef, or high-fat chicken stock as a base; addition of corn syrup or sugar; high sodium content (more than 500 mg per serving)
SALAD	Plenty of mixed greens with any other desired vegetables, such as tomatoes, peppers, snow peas, onions, and cucumbers, and vinaigrette dressing	Salad made with iceberg lettuce, with cheese, croutons, or cold cuts; cream or cheese-based dressing; added salt; large amounts of any oily dressing
SANDWICH	Whole grain bread with no added sugar or fat and limited added salt (less than 1 mg sodium per calorie); lettuce, tomato, and other vegetables or lean, minimally processed meat such as sliced turkey breast; mustard	White bread or any bread with added sugar and fat and/or high sodium content (more than 2 mg per calorie), with mayonnaise, butter, or stick margarine; sliced cheese; processed deli meats, such as bologna, salami, and sausage

2. You learn to shop for and stock your kitchen with simply flavored—but very tasty—foods and ingredients. By the end of the plan, you will use these foods and ingredients to create your own simply flavored meals, which will allow you to go off the meal plan without going off the diet—ever!

The recipes, ingredients, and foods used in the meal plan not only supply your taste buds with the right flavors to subdue your appetite center and induce weight loss, they also have many additional appetite-suppressing and health-promoting properties. For example, the plan's grain products are high in fiber and minimally processed. You'll consume lean meat and dairy products. The sauces, spreads, and dressings are free of trans fats and low in saturated fats.

Before getting started on this delicious new way of eating, however, you need a little background. You'll soon be changing the way you shop, stock your kitchen, cook, and eat. To do that, you need the answers to some important questions. What do you look for on a food label to choose the best, Flavor Point Diet–approved products? What should be in your pantry and refrigerator? How do you address making dietary changes with your teenager? I'll show you.

This knowledge will enable you to apply the benefits of the Flavor Point Diet with maximum flexibility, whatever the composition of your household, whatever ethnic food you prefer, and whatever your income or schedule. This way, you'll have a shortcut to the Flavor Point wherever you go.

THREE PHASES, ONE ULTIMATE GOAL

Depending on your genes, metabolism, and dedication, you'll lose roughly 9 to 16 pounds or more during the next 6 weeks as you progress through the meal plan. After that, as long as you stick with the Flavor Point way of eating, you'll continue to lose weight until you reach your goal.

Phase 1 imposes the greatest degree of dietary discipline, with the later phases a bit less restrictive. Because the Flavor Point Diet is based on the principle of flavor management rather than on cutting foods and food categories out of your diet, everything that helps you lose weight continues as you move from the more restrictive phases to the less restrictive ones. Rather than taking away foods, then adding them back (and doing the same with pounds!), as other diets do, the Flavor Point Diet teaches you to use flavor to organize how you eat in a permanent way. The discipline is more obvious at first, then slowly fades into the background as it becomes part of who you are and how you eat. It never goes away. Rather, it goes from obvious to subtle, from regimented to routine.

The program moves from a *daily flavor theme* in phase 1 to a *meal- and snack-specific flavor theme* in phase 2. After phase 2, you'll no longer need the meal plan. You'll remain on the Flavor Point Plan for life, however, sticking with phase 3 until you reach your weight-loss goal—and forever. In phase 3, the maintenance phase outlined in Chapter 6, you use individual foods to control appetite. From day to meal to food, you will take simple steps toward lifelong mastery of appetite—and permanent weight control!

Flavor Pointer

CEREAL AT THE FLAVOR POINT

Cereal can be one of the best foods you can eat, combining the nutrients and fiber of whole grains with the benefits of the fat-free milk you pour over it and perhaps the fruit you add. That's why the Flavor-Friendly Alternatives in the Flavor Point Meal Plan emphasize breakfast cereal. It's nutritious and filling, especially if you choose the right types.

Some of the best cereals can be a bit pricey. If cost is a factor for you, here's another option. Use any combination of the cooking grains recommended in the meal plan. Make a bit extra when you prepare them for another meal, mix a few varieties together if you like, and— *voilà!*—you have multigrain cereal for pennies a bowl! Eat them plain with milk or sweeten them with a bit of juice or all-fruit preserves, honey, or sugar.

HOW TO USE THE MEAL PLAN

For best results on the Flavor Point Diet, follow these pointers.

- Respect each flavor theme, but feel free to make substitutions using the Flavor-Friendly Alternatives on page 129. In counseling many people who tried many types of diets, I've discovered that few people stick to meal plans. Quite often, dieters look over a meal plan and then alter it to their preferences and lifestyle. In other words, they go on their own version of the plan! In some cases, they still manage to lose weight; in other cases, they don't. Because of this, I've devised a system that allows you to "cheat" and still lose weight. For any breakfast, snack, or lunch item on the menu, you can substitute a Flavor-Friendly Alternative. These items fit into any flavor theme. They're also quick and nearly effortless to prepare. *Note:* One of the flavor-friendly breakfast options is eggs, but you should limit your egg intake to six or fewer per week. Dietary cholesterol is not nearly as harmful as once feared, but too much of almost anything is a bad idea! Also, with the exception of Chow Now options (see page 70), there are no alternatives for dinners and desserts. For these, you must adhere to the plan.

- Refrain from eating fast food during the program. Most fast foods combine the two most addictive flavors—sweet and salty—in one package. If you find you must break this rule (you're at a rest stop in the middle of Nevada, for example, and McDonald's is your only option), break it as gently as possible. Follow the tips for eating out (see page 58) and order a meal that's simple and minimally processed and has few if any flavor additions (such as special sauce). Also, make sure the foods you choose fit into your flavor theme.

- Don't frequent buffet-style restaurants during the program. The human brain is too easily tempted by this type of food variety. Also, most of us tend to justify overeating at an all-you-can-eat buffet because we think it's a bargain. Change your thinking on this. Where's the bargain if, in eating more for free, you gain weight (at no extra charge) that you must later spend money to lose?

● Exercise moderately for 30 minutes most days of the week. Exercise certainly helps with weight loss, and even more with lasting weight control. Equally important, if not more so, it improves your health. Whether you walk, run, cycle, swim, or dance in your bedroom, get some movement into your days. Increase your breathing and heart rate noticeably as you work out, but don't push yourself so hard that you can't talk comfortably in full sentences. You can complete the 30 or more minutes of activity all at once or accumulate that much over the course of the day. Your activity may be exercise, a sport, housework, walking your dog, dancing, or just climbing stairs. The key is to move it if you want to lose it (weight), and gain it (health).

Combine your aerobic activity with resistance training (weight lifting). Resistance exercise—such as lifting weights, pulling against elastic bands, or doing circuit training—builds muscle. Each pound of muscle you build through weight training burns roughly 30 to 50 calories a day, every day. That's right; when you build muscle by working out a few times a week, you burn more calories in your sleep! That's quite a return on investment.

It's never too soon to begin being active, but it's never too late either. Studies of people well into their eighties show clear benefits of physical activity. Start slowly, giving yourself a chance to acclimate. These bodies of ours were made to move, so there's a good chance you'll find physical activity habit forming once you give it a chance.

● Drink roughly six 8-ounce glasses of water throughout the day and have water instead of other beverages, such as soda.

● Whenever possible, finish lunch and dinner with a hot beverage, and sip it slowly. It will help give your brain time to register that you are full and satisfied and will provide a nice sense of closure.

- Always start dinner with a mixed green salad. Rich in nutrients and low in calories, salads turn down your appetite and keep you from overeating other, higher-calorie items.

Your Family at the Flavor Point

FINESSING YOUR ADOLESCENTS

Catherine and I have two adolescents in our home: Rebecca, 17, and Corinda, 16. I have to confess that we encouraged healthful eating before they became teenagers, but if you don't have this same advantage, don't despair!

Adolescents are somewhat autonomous because they're often out of your control and making their own decisions. They also need to push that autonomy to the limits because gaining independence is the very mission of adolescence. Can you respect that and still guide your teens toward the Flavor Point? Absolutely.

First, negotiate. You can find many nutritious substitutes for popular foods that almost all teens will readily accept. To get them to make some changes, allow them to reject others. Show some flexibility.

Set some limits, too, as well as an example. Adolescents are mature enough to deserve some independence but immature enough to need some rules. You do the shopping, after all, so you can agree to still have chips in the house, but you decide which ones.

Be sure not to be judgmental, and certainly don't focus on a child's weight. Rather, make it clear that you care what your teens eat because you care about their health—because you love them! Talk the talk, and make it about love and family solidarity. Walk the walk, so they have an example to follow. Finally, cut them a bit of slack. When you get to the Flavor Point, you'll bump into your teenager, who will try to pretend to be too cool to be seen with you!

- Save alcoholic beverages until near the end of a meal. Although a moderate amount of alcohol is healthful and pleasurable, it lowers your inhibitions, leading to overindulgence. If you wait until the middle or end of the meal, however, you'll circumvent alcohol's appetite-stimulating effect.

- If you decide to have dessert, which is optional in the plan, wait a half hour after dinner. This gives your brain, stomach, and intestines time to communicate your level of fullness. By delaying your gratification, you also enhance the pleasure you get from dessert.

- Use the brands of bread, crackers, and other packaged foods specified in the appendix. I chose these brands for their nutritional value as well as for their availability in regular supermarkets. In some instances, you may have to go to the health food section, but most of the time, you'll find the recommended brands on the regular shelves. These brands have the Flavor Point seal of approval; use others at your own risk!

STOCKING A FLAVOR-FRIENDLY KITCHEN

Before embarking on the meal plan, you need to get your house in order—literally. By buying the following staples and stocking them in your refrigerator, freezer, and pantry, you'll have on hand almost everything you need for the meal plan. The following shopping list remains basically the same from week to week on the plan, so once you get used to buying these ingredients, you'll be able to shop by rote and get through the store faster and faster. Buying the Flavor Point foundation ingredients will become so second nature to you that you'll no longer need to carry a shopping list, and you'll head for all the right aisles without a moment's hesitation! Keep in mind that the suggested amounts of each food are designed to feed a family of four, so adjust how much you buy based on your family's size.

SALAD INGREDIENTS

You'll eat a salad every evening of the week, so get used to having those ingredients in your fridge at all times! Because the following ingredients are prewashed and precut or shredded in resealable packages, you can easily throw handfuls of this and that into a big salad bowl with only minimal rinsing and chopping.

SALAD INGREDIENTS	HOW MUCH?	WHERE IN THE SUPERMARKET?
Alfalfa sprouts	1 box*	Refrigerated produce section
Cherry or grape tomatoes	2 boxes	Refrigerated produce section
Prewashed baby spinach	2 bags*	Refrigerated produce section
Prewashed mixed greens	4 bags*	Refrigerated produce section
Shredded cabbage/carrots	1 bag*	Refrigerated produce section
Shredded carrots	1 bag*	Refrigerated produce section
Shredded red cabbage	1 bag*	Refrigerated produce section

*12–16 oz each

VEGETABLES

You'll need a lot of vegetables each week, as they always accompany the dinner entrée. Whenever you shop, throw fresh or frozen vegetables into your cart. Unless the flavor theme is based on that veggie, feel free to sauté the same amount of whatever veggie you happen to have on hand in the freezer; that way, when you're shopping, you don't have to stop and think what veggies to get. Just get some!

Some of the recipes call for garlic cloves. Buy peeled cloves to save on preparation time and store them in the refrigerator in their original container, tightly closed and placed in a zip-top bag. You'll also occasionally need ginger. Get minced fresh ginger (rather than the dry powder, which isn't as fragrant) to cut preparation time. You can also store fresh ginger in a zip-top bag and grate it as needed. Despite popular belief, you don't

VEGETABLES	HOW MUCH?	WHERE IN THE SUPERMARKET?
Frozen or fresh precut broccoli florets	1 bag	Freezer or produce section
Frozen or fresh precut butternut squash	1 bag	Freezer or produce section
Frozen or fresh cauliflower florets	1 bag	Freezer or produce section
Frozen or fresh string beans	1 bag	Freezer or produce section
Frozen baked fries (Alexia)	1 bag	Freezer section
Frozen chopped onions	1 bag	Freezer section
Frozen corn kernels	1 bag	Freezer or produce section
Frozen peas	1 bag	Freezer section
Frozen precut bell peppers	1 bag	Freezer section
Frozen precut or fresh baby carrots	1 bag	Freezer or produce section
Frozen spinach	2 bags	Freezer section
Minced ginger (or piece of fresh ginger)	1 jar	Refrigerated produce section
Peeled garlic cloves	1 jar	Refrigerated produce section

have to peel it. Although you won't need the Alexia baked fries listed on the opposite page on a regular basis, they keep well and are nutritionally superior to any of the other brands.

GRAINS, LENTILS, AND BEANS

You'll use these staples throughout the meal plan. They have a long shelf life, so have some handy at all times. You'll often find fat-free chicken and vegetable broths in the same aisle, so toss some into the cart to use in soups and stews.

GRAINS, LENTILS, BEANS	HOW MUCH?	WHERE IN THE SUPERMARKET?
Brown rice	1 bag	Rice/soup/dry bean aisle
Bulgur wheat (cracked wheat)*	2 boxes	Rice or cereal aisle
Canned black beans	2 cans	Canned veggie/bean aisle
Canned cannellini beans	2 cans	Canned veggie/bean aisle
Canned chickpeas	2 cans	Canned veggie/bean aisle
Canned ground tomatoes†	2 cans	Pasta/tomato sauce aisle
Canned red beans	2 cans	Canned veggie/bean aisle
Dry lentils	2 bags	Rice/soup/dry bean aisle

*Because this isn't always available in regular supermarkets, you may need to go to a health food store. Buy large amounts in bulk to reduce your trips.

†See the appendix for recommended brands.

(continued)

GRAINS, LENTILS, BEANS *(cont.)*	HOW MUCH?	WHERE IN THE SUPERMARKET?
Dry quinoa	1 bag	Health food aisle
Fat-free chicken or veggie broth	32-oz can	Rice/soup/dry bean aisle
Oat bran flour[†]	1 bag	Baking or health food aisle
Pastry flour[†]	1 bag	Baking or health food aisle
Rolled oats (quick cooking or old fashioned)	1 box	Cereal aisle
7-grain crackers	1 box	Health food or cracker aisle
Whole grain bread[†]	1 bag	Bread aisle
Whole grain cereal[†]	2 boxes	Cereal or health food aisle
Whole grain waffles[†]	1 box	Freezer section or health food aisle
Whole wheat pasta[†]	1 box	Pasta/tomato sauce aisle

*Because this isn't always available in regular supermarkets, you may need to go to a health food store. Buy large amounts in bulk to reduce your trips.

[†]See the appendix for recommended brands.

DAIRY PRODUCTS AND EGGS

You will use fat-free milk and plain yogurt throughout the plan for breakfasts and snacks. You'll also need fat-free buttermilk to thicken sauces and nonfat dry milk as a natural sweetener for baking and as creamer for coffee. Store dry milk in an airtight container or in its original bag. Keep eggs on hand for meals and baking.

DAIRY PRODUCTS AND EGGS	HOW MUCH?	WHERE IN THE SUPERMARKET?
Eggs (organic, with omega-3's)	1/2 doz	Refrigerated dairy section
Fat-free buttermilk	1 qt	Refrigerated dairy section
Fat-free milk	1 gal	Refrigerated dairy section
Fat-free plain yogurt*	32 oz	Refrigerated dairy section
Nonfat dry milk	1 box	Coffee/tea aisle

*See the appendix for recommended brands.

LEAN PROTEIN

Keep a package of chicken cutlets (about 1 pound) and a package of tilapia fillets (about 1 pound) in your freezer to use at the last minute on a Chow Now day (you'll learn more about these special days in Chapter 4). If you can't find skinless chicken pieces at your supermarket, ask the person at the meat counter to remove the skin; there's no extra charge. Freeze the extra-lean ground turkey and use it as needed. Also keep frozen shrimp on hand at all times; it's used in several of the recipes.

LEAN PROTEIN	HOW MUCH?	WHERE IN THE SUPERMARKET?
Extra-lean ground turkey	1 lb	Refrigerated meat section
Frozen raw easy-peel shrimp	1 bag	Freezer fish section
Skinless chicken cutlets	4 (4 oz each)	Refrigerated meat section
Tilapia fillets	4 (4–5 oz each)	Refrigerated meat or seafood section

MISCELLANEOUS

Keep the following items on hand for cooking or baking. You'll use them occasionally throughout the Flavor Point Meal Plan.

MISCELLANEOUS INGREDIENTS	HOW MUCH?	WHERE IN THE SUPERMARKET?
All-fruit jam or preserves*	1 jar	Jarred food aisle
Almonds	1 bag	Baking aisle
Applesauce (unsweetened)	1 jar	Canned fruit and juice aisle
Balsamic vinegar	1 bottle	Condiment/dressing aisle
Basil pesto*	1 container	Refrigerated section
Canned peaches (in pear juice)	2 cans (4 oz each)	Canned fruit and juice aisle
Canned pineapple (in juice)	2 cans (4 oz each)	Canned fruit and juice aisle
Canola oil	1 bottle	Condiment/dressing aisle
Dijon mustard	1 jar	Condiment/dressing aisle
Dried fruit (currants/ raisins, cranberries, prunes, etc.)	As needed	Canned fruit and juice aisle
Dry spices	As needed	Baking aisle
Flax meal and/or flaxseed (refrigerate after opening)	1 bag	Health food aisle
Fresh fruit	As needed	Produce section
Fresh vegetables	As needed	Produce section
Honey	1 jar	Baking aisle
Hummus* (plain)	1 jar	Refrigerated section

MISCELLANEOUS INGREDIENTS *(cont.)*	HOW MUCH?	WHERE IN THE SUPERMARKET?
Margarine (trans-fat-free)*	1 container	Refrigerated dairy aisle
Natural almond butter	1 container	Health food aisle
Natural peanut butter	1 container	Bread aisle
Newman's Own Light Italian Dressing†	1 bottle	Condiment/dressing aisle
Nuts/seeds	As needed	Baking aisle
Olive oil (extra virgin)	1 bottle	Condiment/dressing aisle
Orange juice concentrate	1 container	Freezer section
Pineapple juice concentrate	1 container	Freezer section
Salsa, mild*	1 jar	Condiment/dressing aisle

*See the appendix for recommended brands.

†A 16-ounce bottle of dressing should last you about 2 weeks, depending on whether you also use it for your flavor-friendly lunch salad.

READING FOOD LABELS FOR FLAVOR

Now that you know what types of foods to buy, it's time to talk about choosing the best brands, especially of packaged foods. In every food category, from bread to barbecue sauce, you can choose from better brands and worse brands (see the appendix for a comprehensive list of my favorites). To choose the best brands consistently, you must learn how to read the fine print on food labels.

To interpret a food label with minimal effort, follow this general rule: For every 100-calorie serving of a packaged food, the amount of sodium should be less than 1.5 milligrams per calorie, fat should be 3 or fewer grams, added sugars should be 3 or fewer grams, and fiber should be more than 2 grams. If, for example, a 110-calorie serving of a food

(continued on page 58)

Which Label Is Flavor Friendly?

Below, you'll find the Nutrition Facts panel and ingredients list from a leading breakfast cereal.

1. Often, the Nutrition Facts pertain to just a portion of the contents. A serving may have 100 calories, but if there are 2.5 servings per package, the entire package has 250 calories.

2. Calories count! This is the number of calories per serving, so pay attention to serving size. Calories come from protein (4 calories per gram), carbohydrate (4 calories per gram), and fat (9 calories per gram).

3. Both the total amount and type of fat are important. Avoid foods with saturated and trans fats.

4. Fiber is your friend! It helps you reach the Flavor Point faster. Whole grains provide it in abundance; refined grains do not.

5. This may look impressive, but it generally means that the equivalent of a multivitamin was mixed into the ingredients. Such fortification adds valuable nutrients, but you can obtain these same nutrients from a vitamin pill instead.

6. The ingredients list is separate from but usually printed near the Nutrition Facts label. It lists ingredients in order of abundance. In other words, packaged foods contain more of the ingredients near the beginning of the list and less of those near the end.

Nutrition Facts

Serving Size: 1 cup (30g)
Servings Per Container: About 17

Amount Per Serving	Cereal	with ½ cup skim milk
Calories	110	150
Calories from fat	10	10
	% Daily Value†	
Total Fat 1g*	1%	2%
Saturated fat 0g	0%	0%
Polyunsaturated fat 0g		
Monounsaturated fat 0g		
Cholesterol 0mg	0%	1%
Sodium 220mg	9%	12%
Potassium 105mg	3%	9%
Total Carbohydrate 24g	8%	10%
Dietary fiber 3g	13%	13%
Sugars 4g		
Other carbohydrate 17g		
Protein 3g		
Vitamin A	10%	15%
Vitamin C	10%	10%
Calcium	2%	15%
Iron	45%	45%
Vitamin D	10%	25%
Thiamin	50%	50%
Riboflavin	50%	60%
Niacin	50%	50%
Vitamin B$_6$	50%	50%
Folic Acid	50%	50%
Vitamin B$_{12}$	50%	60%
Phosphorus	10%	20%
Magnesium	8%	10%
Zinc	50%	50%
Copper	4%	4%

*Amount in cereal. A serving of cereal plus skim milk provides 1g total fat, less than 5mg cholesterol, 280mg sodium, 310mg potassium, 30g total carbohydrate (10g sugars) and 7g protein.

†Percent Daily Values are based on a 2,000-calorie diet. Your Daily Values may be higher or lower depending on your calorie needs.

	Calories:	2,000	2,500
Total Fat	Less than	65g	80g
Sat Fat	Less than	20g	25g
Cholesterol	Less than	300mg	300mg
Sodium	Less than	2,400mg	2,400mg
Potassium		3,500mg	3,500mg
Total Carbohydrate		300g	375g
Dietary Fiber		25g	30g

INGREDIENTS: Whole wheat, sugar, salt, corn syrup, partially hydrogenated soybean oil, brown sugar syrup, natural flavor, trisodium phosphate, freshness preserved by BHT.

VITAMINS AND MINERALS: Zinc and iron (mineral nutrients), a B vitamin (niacinamide), vitamin C (sodium ascorbate), vitamin B$_6$ (pyridoxine hydrochloride), vitamin B$_2$ (riboflavin), vitamin B$_1$ (thiamin mononitrate), vitamin A (palmitate), a B vitamin (folic acid), vitamin B$_{12}$, vitamin D.

Below, you'll find the Nutrition Facts panel and ingredient list from Nature's Path Organic Multigrain Oat Bran Flakes, a brand recommended in the Flavor Point Diet.

1. This minimally processed food contains no trans fat.

2. Note that even this cereal contains both sugar and salt, but at much lower levels than are available in most commercial brands.

3. Natural, unprocessed grains provide an excellent source of fiber.

4. These nutrients are naturally present in the food, not added in at the end.

5. This ingredient list is rather long, but only because the cereal is made from multiple whole grains. There are no artificial ingredients, no flavor enhancers, and no chemicals. The only chemical-sounding names you ever want to see on an ingredients list refer to added vitamins and minerals. Otherwise, accept a product with a long ingredients list only if all of the listings describe foods and ingredients you recognize, such as several whole grains in a multigrain bread or cereal.

Nutrition Facts

Serving Size: ¾ cup (30g)
Servings Per Container: About 12

Amount Per Serving	Cereal	Cereal + 125 ml of fortified skim milk
Calories	**110**	**150**
Calories from fat	10	10
	% Daily Value†	
Total Fat 1g*	**2%**	**2%**
Saturated fat 0g	0%	0%
Trans fat 0g	0%	0%
Cholesterol 0mg	**0%**	**1%**
Sodium 115mg	**5%**	**8%**
Total Carbohydrate 24g	**8%**	**10%**
Dietary fiber 5g	20%	20%
Sugars 4g		
Protein 4g		
Vitamin A	0%	6%
Vitamin C	0%	0%
Calcium	2%	15%
Iron	10%	10%

*Amount in cereal. One-half cup of skim milk contributes an additional 40 calories, 65mg sodium, 6g total carbohydrates (6g sugars) and 4g protein.

†Percent Daily Values are based on a 2,000-calorie diet. Your Daily Values may be higher or lower depending on your calorie needs.

	Calories:	2,000	2,500
Total Fat	Less than	65g	80g
Sat Fat	Less than	20g	25g
Cholesterol	Less than	300mg	300mg
Sodium	Less than	2,400mg	2,400mg
Potassium		3,500mg	3,500mg
Total Carbohydrate		300g	375g
Dietary Fiber		25g	30g

Calories per gram: Fat 9 • Carbohydrate 4 • Protein 4

INGREDIENTS: Organic whole oat flour, organic whole wheat flour, organic wheat bran, organic evaporated cane juice, organic oat bran, organic yellow cornmeal, organic brown rice flour, organic barley malt extract, sea salt, organic whole wheat sprouts.

provides 220 milligrams of sodium, it's too salty! This is okay if it's supposed to be a salty food, but certainly not if it's breakfast cereal!

In addition to that general rule, follow these pointers.

- Try not to buy packaged foods that include trans fat (partially hydrogenated oil) on the list of ingredients.
- Avoid buying packaged foods that have high-fructose corn syrup on the ingredient list. This is a long-winded way of saying "added sugars."
- Choose foods with short ingredient lists. This is crucial. Generally, the longer the ingredient list, the more the food has been processed, and the more unnecessary flavors it contains. Wholesome, minimally processed foods with simple, uncluttered flavors tend to have short ingredient lists. One exception is foods made from multiple whole grains, but you'll soon learn to tell the difference.

To practice your label-reading skills, consider the two ingredient labels on pages 56 and 57. Of the two, the Nature's Path cereal is a clear winner over its mainstream counterpart. The popular commercial cereal has less fiber and more sodium, trans fats, corn syrup, and flavor enhancers. True, the equivalent of a multivitamin is thrown in for good measure, but if you want a multivitamin, take one—and then eat a wholesome, minimally processed cereal for breakfast!

STAYING ON POINT IN RESTAURANTS

Ideally, you'll cook most of your Flavor Point meals at home. That said, let's be realistic. Everyone goes out to eat from time to time. I know—we do it, too!

When you eat out, either order dishes that match the flavor theme of the day or choose dishes that resemble the Flavor-Friendly Alternatives (see page 129). I recommend that you avoid eating out during phase 1 of the meal plan, when you're maintaining a daylong flavor theme. You'll

Your Restaurant Survival Guide

Use these pointers when eating at the following types of restaurants.

ITALIAN: Choose pasta, fish, seafood, or poultry dishes with tomato-, olive oil-, or wine-based sauces. Avoid excessive cheese, cream sauces, or meat.

ASIAN: Choose vegetarian, tofu, seafood, and poultry dishes. Ask for low-oil preparation.

MEXICAN: Avoid fried items, including tortilla chips, and dishes with excessive cheese. Choose soft tortillas instead of hard taco shells. Ask for fat-free refried beans.

FRENCH: Avoid dishes with excessive cream, butter, or cheese. Select restaurants offering southern French, or Provençal, cooking, which tends to be much lighter than northern French cuisine.

DELIS: Choose whole grain breads and lean cold cuts such as sliced turkey breast. Avoid fatty, highly processed meats such as pastrami and corned beef. Use mustard instead of butter or mayonnaise.

GRILLS AND DINERS: Avoid fried foods and burgers. Take advantage of the wide selection to choose salads (avoid cheese and croutons), vegetable side dishes, fish, poultry, pasta, or vegetarian dishes.

more easily fit restaurant meals into the plan during phases 2 and 3. Going out to eat is fine, but going off the plan is not, because if you do, you of course lose some of its benefits!

Try to choose restaurants that:

• Offer a variety of dishes made with whole grain products (such as pasta), fish, seafood, vegetables, and poultry.

- Are willing to modify dishes to suit your preferences.
- Indicate nutritious, low-calorie/low-fat, or heart-healthy choices on the menu.
- Offer a variety of vegetable salads.
- Tend to use low-fat sauces, such as vinaigrettes, wine sauces, citrus-juice sauces, and tomato sauces.
- Provide adequate but not excessive portions. Refer to the portion sizes given throughout the meal plan for an idea of what reasonable portions look like.

Avoid restaurants that:

- Serve only or mostly fried food.
- Won't modify dishes to suit your preferences.
- Use mostly cream- or cheese-based sauces.
- Offer buffets or all-you-can-eat options.
- Provide especially large portions.
- Don't offer nutritious, heart-healthy, or low-calorie/low-fat options on the menu.

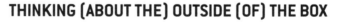
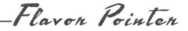

THINKING (ABOUT THE) OUTSIDE (OF) THE BOX

It's bad enough that a highly processed food supply bombards us with an excess of flavors that push the Flavor Point into outer space, along with an excess of sugar, saturated fat, trans fats, and salt. Adding insult to injury, most food packaging is deceptive! Bold claims on the front about health effects and nutrient composition are all too often belied by the facts on the back! Don't be suckered by front-of-the-box sales pitches. Look for the ingredients list and the Nutrition Facts panel, and judge your food by what's actually in it.

Once you're inside the restaurant and seated at the table, you can take additional steps to stay on point. When the server comes to your table, ask the following questions.

1. Do you have any healthful dishes to recommend?
2. Does the menu give complete information about what's in a dish?
3. Is the chef/cook willing to modify dishes to make them healthier?

Then, before ordering any item from the menu, ask the server:

1. What's in the sauce of this dish? Does it contain butter, cream, or cheese?
2. Is this dish rich or light in your opinion?
3. Are there any ingredients in this dish not listed on the menu, such as cream, cheese, or meat?

STAYING ON POINT AT FAST-FOOD RESTAURANTS

I'd like to tell you to stop eating fast food altogether. Most fast-food restaurants offer selections that are very high in fat and calories, high in saturated fat and trans fat, high in sugar or salt, and very limited in nutritional value. Most of their options combine too many flavors and calories in small packages. They are not flavor friendly!

That said, fast-food restaurants are convenient and inexpensive, and you may find them irresistible from time to time. Even as you work to reduce the role of fast food in your diet, use the following tips to improve the choices you make.

- Choose franchises such as Subway that offer and identify nutritious dishes instead of franchises that specialize in burgers or fried foods.
- Don't order deep-fried foods.
- At any fast-food restaurant or franchise you intend to visit repeatedly, ask to see a chart showing the calorie and nutritional content of the

dishes you order. (You can find the nutritional composition of foods at leading fast-food restaurants at www.fatcalories.com.) Identify and stick with minimally processed items with the fewest unnecessary additions of flavor enhancers. For example, a plain burger is better than a bacon cheeseburger smeared with mystery sauce.

- Don't order large or super sizes. These may give you more food for your dollar, but they also provide more calories, more fat, more salt, and more sugar than any human being could possibly need in a meal.
- Choose water instead of soda. Sodas add many empty calories to a meal as well as increase the variety of flavors.
- Always make a salad with low-fat dressing part of your meal.
- Always add extra vegetables (such as sliced lettuce, tomato, and onion) to your meal.
- Refrain from additions such as cheese or bacon.
- Choose dishes that are grilled, baked, broiled, or poached. Also look for lean meat, fish, vegetarian, and heart-healthy options.

STAYING ON POINT AT WORK

Don't let your company's cafeteria or vending machine options dictate how well you stick to the Flavor Point Meal Plan. Instead, get into the habit of using an insulated lunch bag to take nutritious lunch and snack items with you to work each day. This needn't take a lot of time. Consider the following quick and easy options.

Whole grain cereal. Pick a whole grain cereal from the recommended list in the appendix and pack ½ cup in a large zip-top bag to have as a morning snack. Either munch on it plain or mix it with fat-free yogurt. Don't pack most major brands of cereal-and-milk bars, breakfast bars, or muffin bars. Although they claim to be whole grain cereal, in fact, they're nothing more than candy filled with sugar, salt, hydrogenated oils, and flavor enhancers.

Fresh fruit. Refreshing, sweet, relatively low in calories, and generally

Your Family at the Flavor Point

BETWIXT WITH TWEENS

If you have children between the ages of 10 and 13, you have tweens! Congratulations. We have them, too. Two, in fact: Valerie, age 11, and Natalia, age 10.

Tweens are still very dependent on you for their food choices; they can't just take off to McDonald's with their friends. That said, they are certainly old enough to have strong opinions. To take them to the Flavor Point, follow these tips.

- Give your kids an active voice in food selection. The more involved they are, the more cooperative they will be.
- If possible, let them help with food preparation. Tweens are much more willing to try a new food if they've had a hand in its preparation.
- Ask them to try the same new food repeatedly to give them a chance to acclimate to it.

The Flavor Point Meal Plan will ease the way. Some of our pilot study participants told me that their kids had never really liked their cooking until they started following the Flavor Point Diet. Don't leave your children behind, betwixt, and between. Take them by the hand and set them securely on the path to the Flavor Point right along with you.

rich in both nutrients and fiber, just about all types of fresh fruit make great snacks or accompaniments to lunch. Wash and cut or section fruit in advance so it's ready to eat. Match the fruit to the flavor theme of the day during phases 1 and 2 and stick to one fruit at a time for phase 3.

Dried fruit. Choose fruits that contain no added oils or sugar. Dates, figs, raisins, apricots, pears, prunes, and dried bananas taste as sweet and chewy as candy but are great sources of nutrients, vitamins, and fiber. Match the dried fruit with the theme of the day in phases 1 and 2 and stick with one type at a time for phase 3.

Canned fruit. Fruit packed in natural fruit juices is convenient to carry. Don't buy fruit packed in any kind of syrup, even light syrup. Unsweetened applesauce is also delicious and convenient. It's available in different flavor combinations, such as apricot, berries, or cinnamon, and can match a particular theme during any phase of the plan. Stay away from so-called fruit snacks in the form of little gummy characters, rollups, or "gushers." They offer no nutrition and lots of added sugar, dyes, and flavor enhancers. If you must indulge your sweet tooth, Stretch Island 100% Organic Fruit Leather fits into the plan. These flat bars are actually concentrated fruit with no added sugar or oils.

Yogurt. Fat-free plain or fruit yogurt makes a great snack. Combine

Your Family at the Flavor Point

PACIFYING YOUR PIPSQUEAKS

I have been surprised at the number of times parents have told me their 3- or 4-year-olds simply refuse to eat the right foods. What would you do if your child simply refused not to play in traffic?

To encourage your young children to eat healthier foods, be assertive. How your kids eat is every bit as important to their health as being vaccinated or getting enough exercise. Second, keep trying. Familiarity breeds preference! We all like what we're used to, and your children will dislike new foods just because they are new. Stick with them for a while. Once your chil-

dren adjust, they'll be much more accepting.

Third, no one, including a child, likes to be duped. Your kids will doubtless want the products they see peddled on TV. As soon as they're old enough to understand (our 6-year-old son certainly is), tell them that food ads may be deceiving them into eating things that really aren't good for them.

Discuss, explain, set limits, occasionally compromise, and, above all, set a good example. Your child will follow you toward a lifetime of health. There is no greater gift a parent can give!

½ cup with dried fruit, fresh fruit, and/or cereal, and you have a meal! Yogurt provides plenty of calcium and is convenient to carry in single-serving containers. Check the serving size on packaged yogurt to make sure you're getting only ½ cup.

Whole grain or multigrain bread. Pick from the list of recommended whole grain breads in the appendix and use two slices to create your own signature flavor-friendly sandwiches. If you opt for a brand not listed in the appendix, make sure it has at least 2 grams of fiber per 100 calories and no trans fats (partially hydrogenated oil) or high-fructose corn syrup.

Whole grain crackers. Pick from the following list of whole grain crackers. Spread the recommended amount with 2 tablespoons of hummus for an afternoon snack. If you opt for other brands, make sure they have at least 2 grams of fiber per 100 calories.

2 Ak-Mak 100% Whole Wheat Sesame Crackers
10 GeniSoy Deep Sea Salt Soy Crisps
5 Kashi TLC Original 7-Grain Crackers
5 Old London Whole Wheat Melba Snacks
3 Old London Whole Wheat Melba Toasts
6 Snyder's of Hanover Oat Bran Sticks
4 Stacy's Simply Naked Baked Pita Chips
2 Wasa Light Rye or Hearty Rye Crispbreads

Veggies. Crunchy and satisfying to chew, raw vegetables are generally very low in calories and high in nutrients and fiber. Choose from convenient prewashed, packaged veggies in the produce section, such as baby carrots, broccoli, cauliflower, and green beans. Eat them plain or with fat-free yogurt dips from the meal plan, or try dipping them in store-bought hummus, fat-free bean dip, or fat-free salsa that you've packed in a small container. Consider purchasing a special container designed to hold a salad and a specific amount of dressing. Put packaged grated carrots, coleslaw, or broccoli and baby spinach and other greens in the bottom section and fill the top with 2 capfuls of Newman's Own Light Italian Dressing.

Dips. For a great afternoon snack, take along some dip and whole grain bread, crackers, or veggies. Make your own dips from beans or veggies or buy prepared dips, hummus, salsa, or fat-free cottage cheese or yogurt (consult the appendix for recommended brands).

Nuts and seeds. Packed with healthful essential natural oils, dry-roasted or raw nuts make a convenient snack food. Because they're easy to overeat, however, pack only a small portion and take along only one variety per day. You can also buy packaged trail mixes, which are combinations of dried fruits, nuts, seeds, and cereals, but avoid mixes that include any added sugar or oil, coconut, or chocolate chips.

Lean protein. Use the following lean protein foods for your lunches.

3 ounces water-packed light tuna in a pouch or can

1 hard-cooked egg packed in a zip-top bag

⅓ cup rinsed and drained chickpeas or beans mixed with salad greens packed in a bag or container

3 slices plain, unprocessed roasted turkey breast packed in a zip-top bag

Drinks. Always take a bottle filled with ice water. Don't pack sports drinks, juice cocktails, or sodas.

PART 2

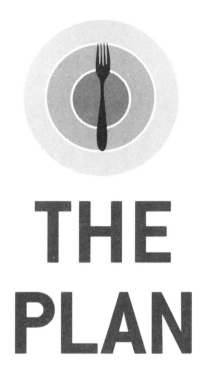

THE
PLAN

THE FLAVOR POINT
MEAL PLAN

6 weeks of delicious, convenient, and flavor-
friendly meals that turn down the Flavor Point.

Are you a busy parent who sometimes doesn't have time to microwave a frozen dinner, much less pull out the pots and pans and become reacquainted with your oven? Have you always wanted to lose weight but just couldn't find the internal motivation, energy, and time to pull it off?

Even if you answered yes to both questions, you can still succeed on the Flavor Point Diet. A busy mother of five developed and tested all of the recipes in this meal plan. With a 6-year-old in first grade and taking Tae Kwon Do and soccer, a 10- and 11-year-old needing help with homework and rides to dance classes, two teens with active social lives, three dogs, two rabbits, and me to look after, my wife and writing partner, Catherine doesn't exactly have spare time on her hands! Over the years, she's developed many timesaving tricks that help her create delicious, mouthwatering, healthful and *convenient* meals night after night after night. She buys prechopped vegetables, has developed many quick-prep cooking techniques, and has learned to always have all the right ingredients at hand.

She shares those timesaving tricks with you throughout this meal plan and in the recipes in Chapter 5. In less time than it would take to get to and from the drive-thru, you can prepare a Flavor Point Diet meal!

Whenever possible, we suggest breakfasts, lunches, and snacks that require minimal preparation. Although dinners require slightly more prep work, these too will become a convenient way of life once you properly stock your kitchen and begin to make certain meals and side dishes by rote. In our test group, we found that most participants were able to significantly decrease their prep time by week 2.

Unlike many meal plans you may find in other diet books, this one also offers you plenty of choices. You can follow the standard plan, sticking to each suggested breakfast, lunch, dinner, and snack exactly. Or you can go off the beaten path slightly, depending on your goals. Let's say you'd like to lose weight more quickly. Perhaps your high school reunion is coming up, and you want to look your best. In the meal plan, you'll find suggestions to make that happen. Or maybe you've had a busy week and haven't had time to shop for food. Not to worry. The plan includes emergency rations that you can turn to when you're crunched for time.

The more you make the plan fit your needs, the more successful you'll become. If you find a meal you particularly like or one you don't like, go ahead and replace that meal with another from the same week. It's that flexible. Every dieter I've ever counseled has changed the diet plan they were on to suit their particular needs. Since I know you're just as likely to modify this meal plan, I've built in tips for doing so right from the start. Let's take a look at how the plan allows you to customize it to your needs.

 ## CHOW NOW MEALS

Most Flavor Point Diet dinners are simple and relatively quick to prepare, but some of them do require time to cook or bake—from 15 minutes to 1 hour (in the case of roast chicken). On days when you know you're going to walk in the door at 7 in the evening, and the whole family is going to want "chow now," we designed 1 or 2 days per week where dinner requires 15 minutes or less, including cooking time, from start to finish. That's probably less time than it takes to get to a fast-food restaurant, which is why I like to call these Chow Now meals. Plan on these dinners for days when you know you'll be busy.

You don't need to follow the exact sequence of the meal plan; you simply must stick with the choices for that week. Thus, if you have a busy day on a Wednesday, but you see a meal with a Chow Now symbol on a Tuesday, go ahead and cook Tuesday's suggested meal on Wednesday! If you plan ahead, you can save even more time. For example, when you prepare any dinner, make twice as much and use the leftovers later in the week. Do that twice in a week, and you'll cut out 2 days of food preparation! You may find that preparing dinners on the weekend and having them handy in the refrigerator or freezer to repeat on a busy day during the week also works well.

SPECIAL INDULGENCE DAYS

At the end of the meal plan, you will find two special days, one based on chocolate and the other on coconut. Yummy, right? Even these indulgences are Flavor Point approved and wonderfully nutritious. Any time during or after week 3 of the plan, you can select up to one indulgence day per week.

Our group of 20 men and women who tested the meal plan loved these meals and turned to them regularly. The chocolate lovers in particular told me that the indulgence days were a great aspect of this diet because eating their favorite flavor repeatedly on just one day during the week subdued their cravings for that flavor the rest of the week. So don't feel guilty. Just indulge!

FLAVOR-FRIENDLY ALTERNATIVES

Many nutritious foods, such as whole grain breakfast cereals, are relatively flavor neutral and fit into any flavor theme. In addition to cereal, fresh fruits and vegetables work for any phase of any week of the meal plan. I've included a list of flavor-friendly options, which you can mix and match with any flavor theme, on page 129. This provides you with more control over your daily menu, more choices, and more convenience. All of the Flavor-Friendly Alternatives require little or no preparation and no special shopping, and they even adapt to restaurant eating. For example, when you're eating out for breakfast, pick the cereal option with fat-free milk, the whole grain toast, the oatmeal, or two eggs. When eating lunch at a restaurant, you can choose the salad with oil and vinegar on the side and grilled fish or chicken breast. Just stick with the amount specified in the menu plan. You can use these options at any time for any meal during any week or phase of the plan.

⟨≡WLE   WEIGHT-LOSS EXPRESS

The Flavor Point Diet will help you lose weight at a brisk but reasonable pace and then help you keep it off forever. When I tested the diet on 20 participants, however, I learned that for some people, the meal plan provides more food than they need to feel full and satisfied. If you fall into that category, don't try to stuff yourself silly in order to lose weight! If you wouldn't mind cutting a few more calories and losing weight even faster, use the Weight-Loss Express options. You can make these lower-calorie substitutions for various meals throughout the plan; just look for the symbol.

THE FAMILY PLAN

Any weight-loss program is designed especially for the person who is trying to lose weight—you! If you have a family, you know how difficult it is to go on a diet while serving different food to everyone else. The Flavor Point Meal Plan will help you avoid this problem. Catherine tested all of her recipes on our family of seven people, including children ranging from age 6 to age 17. Also, during our pilot test of the diet, participants took their whole families along with them and reported that, for the most part, their spouses and kids loved the food! We have incredible reports of spouses and children losing weight (sometimes as much as or more than the actual dieter!) and improving their health. If, however, your children object to certain meals on the plan, look to the Flavor-Friendly Alternatives for help. Make these quick and easy meals for your children and something more adult and delicious for yourself.

To make the plan as family friendly as possible, most dinners serve four unless otherwise noted. If you have fewer people to feed, either prepare single servings or freeze the leftovers for a meal later during the week or for other phases of the plan. Every recipe in the plan will be just as delicious after spending a few weeks in your freezer.

As with dinner, desserts also always serve four (and sometimes six). Dessert is, of course, optional, but it's available on every day of the plan, and the nutritional analysis you'll find at the bottom of each daily menu always includes dessert. Feel free to indulge if you need something sweet to end your meal or as an evening snack. You can, of course, omit dessert to accelerate your weight loss.

(continued on page 76)

Can You Drink Coffee?

Although some diets recommend that you cut back on caffeine in order to lose weight, I don't see any need for this. First, going without caffeine may make you tired, and if you're tired, you'll have more difficulty sticking with your new habits. Second, research shows that caffeine probably facilitates weight loss. So there's no need to give up that morning cup of Joe! Just be careful what you put in it, since the calories in sugar and cream can quickly add up. That's why I recommend using undiluted nonfat dry milk (unlike liquid fat-free milk, it won't turn your coffee gray).

Satisfaction at the Flavor Point

THE FLAVOR FACTS

Name: Patty Finn

Age: 45

Hometown: Ansonia, Connecticut

Family status: Single

Occupation: Assistant director of economic development for Derby, Connecticut

Starting weight: 234

Pounds lost: 24 in 12 weeks

Health stats: Blood pressure dropped 21 points; cholesterol dropped 24 points; lost 7 inches from waist; over 7 percent decline in body fat

---

"My slip fell down at work again today. I reached up for something, and it fell right down to the floor. That's a good thing. It fell down because I lost 24 pounds! Until I have a chance to go out and get some new ones, I guess I'll just have to safety-pin my slips to my skirts!

"I've struggled with fad diets in the past. I tried low-carb diets, and I'm not a meat eater, so I just found them to be gross. Then I tried xenadrine supplements to boost my me-

tabolism. They turned me into a total monster. I lost weight fast with both plans, but when I stopped them, the pounds came back twofold.

"I knew of Dr. Katz and was very impressed with what I had heard about him, so I knew his plan was probably not only effective but also realistic and healthy. I went for it.

"I think the most important thing Dr. Katz taught, which I'll take with me for life, is to examine what I'm eating, to take a box and read every ingredient that I'm putting in my body. Before this plan, I was constantly on the run, so I often ate things that were quick . . . and not so good for me. I'm still just as busy, but Dr. Katz has shown me how to make better choices. For instance, he taught me that even though the packaging leads unsuspecting customers (like me) to believe they're healthful, cereal bars are loaded with sugar. He taught me a quick and easy way to choose better foods: Look at the list of ingredients on the box. The fewer ingredients listed, the more nutritious and less appetite-stimulating the food.

"I also think the plan worked well for me because it incorporated foods I like. There is nothing in it that I got sick of. Whenever a sweet tooth strikes, I now have healthful foods I can eat to satisfy it. Plus, I now enjoy sitting down for a good meal instead of constantly eating on the go.

"For breakfast and lunch, I usually chose one of the flavor-friendly options, like cereal or a salad with chicken breast or soup. For dinner, I loved the chicken dishes. I'm a chicken person. My favorite dish was the Roast Chicken with Currant Wine Glaze and Caramelized Onions.

"As far as the snacks are concerned, I've never been a big snacker. Most of the time, I don't even eat the snacks—or the desserts—because I'm too full. There is almost too much food on the program; I can't finish it all.

"Overall, I can honestly say my food preferences have changed. Now I look at a plate of fries, and I don't want them anymore.

"When I'm eating out, I now truly see that restaurant portions are at least three times too big. When I go out to a restaurant, I ask for foods to be grilled instead of fried, and I never finish my whole meal.

"One of the best outcomes of the program is that I no longer take my prescription medication for heartburn. I haven't had heartburn at all since I started the program 12 weeks ago! I've also noticed that my energy level has gone through the roof, and I've been walking every morning as a result.

"People have really noticed my weight loss and have been encouraging me. My boyfriend works out a lot and watches what he eats. He was happy that I tried Dr. Katz's program instead of yet another fad diet—he wants me to lose weight sensibly and healthfully, and that's exactly what this program has helped me to do.

"I will most definitely stay on Dr. Katz's program. I will never ever go back to the weight I was at before I started. This program makes complete sense, and I'm sticking with it for life!" ■

LEARNING BY ROTE

Each dinner in the plan includes a source of protein along with the following quick and easy staples. If, some evening, you find yourself with absolutely no time to make dinner, you can throw a nutritious meal together for the whole family by grabbing a ready-made roast chicken at your local supermarket and serving it (without the skin) with the salad, whole grain, and veggies below in less than 5 minutes.

Salad. Every day with dinner, you'll have a salad, something you throw together without even a thought. To make this truly effortless, keep packaged, prewashed baby greens and precut veggies in your fridge, ready to go every day. Just mix with olive oil and vinegar or Newman's Own Light Italian Dressing.

Bulgur wheat. With almost every dinner, you'll make a whole grain side dish. Bulgur wheat, or cracked wheat, is a great choice. This delicious whole grain side dish takes 5 minutes to prepare, and it will become a hit with your kids. It's relatively low in calories and high in fiber and protein. It also never clumps. Double the recipe and keep leftovers handy to use cold for a lunch salad. You can also reheat it for 2 minutes in the microwave for a subsequent dinner side dish. Bulgur keeps well for 1 week in an airtight container in the fridge.

Vegetables. You'll also have veggies every evening, either as part of the sauce for the main entrée or separately, sautéed in olive oil. Feel free to use packaged, precut vegetables, either frozen or fresh. The recipe for sautéing is always the same: Heat 1 to 2 teaspoons of olive oil in a skillet on high heat, add the veggies, a pinch of salt, and cook for 5 minutes. That's it! Unless the flavor theme is based on a particular vegetable, feel free to sauté the same amount of whatever veggies you happen to have on hand. That way, you don't have to stop and think about which veggies to get when shopping.

PHASE 1

WEEK 1

DAY 1 **RAISIN/CURRANT DAY**

DAY 2 **PINEAPPLE DAY**

DAY 3 **CRANBERRY DAY**

DAY 4 **LEMON DAY**

DAY 5 **PEACH DAY**

DAY 6 **ORANGE DAY**   CN

DAY 7 **APPLE DAY**

DAY 1 **RAISIN/CURRANT DAY**

BREAKFAST

1 cup whole grain cereal (such as Nature's Path Heritage) with 2 Tbsp raisins and ½ cup fat-free milk

OR

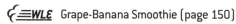 Grape-Banana Smoothie (page 150)

MIDMORNING SNACK

1 cup fat-free plain yogurt with 1 Tbsp raisins or currants

LUNCH

Currant-Lentil Spinach Salad with Feta and Walnuts (page 168)

MIDAFTERNOON SNACK

Grape-Banana Smoothie (page 150)

OR

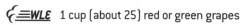 1 cup (about 25) red or green grapes

DINNER FOR 4

Roast Chicken with Currant Wine Glaze and Caramelized Onions (page 188)

1 lb sautéed fresh or frozen green beans

Tossed Garden Salad (page 211; add 1 Tbsp currants)

DESSERT FOR 4 (OPTIONAL)

Raisin-Granola Parfait (page 240)

OR

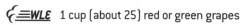 1 cup (about 25) red or green grapes

*See the appendix for other Flavor Point–friendly alternatives.

Daily Nutrition Facts

REGULAR

1,499 calories: 19% from fat (3% from sat fat), 25% from protein, 54% from carbohydrate; 30 g fiber, 173 mg cholesterol, 1,850 mg sodium

WEIGHT-LOSS EXPRESS

1,301 calories: 21% from fat (4% from sat fat), 23% from protein, 53% from carbohydrate; 23 g fiber, 166 mg cholesterol, 1,423 mg sodium

DAY 2 **PINEAPPLE DAY**

BREAKFAST

1 cup whole grain cereal with $^1/_2$ cup fat-free milk

$^3/_4$ cup 100% pineapple juice

OR

WLE Pineapple Smoothie (page 151)

MIDMORNING SNACK

$^3/_4$ cup low-fat pineapple yogurt

LUNCH

Pineapple-Walnut Chicken Salad (page 177)

5 Kashi TLC Original 7-Grain Crackers

MIDAFTERNOON SNACK

$^1/_2$ cup fresh or canned unsweetened pineapple chunks

OR

WLE 10 oz pineapple fizz (6 oz seltzer water and 4 oz 100% pineapple juice)

DINNER FOR 4

Pineapple Shrimp (page 210)

4 cups cooked bulgur wheat (page 228)

1 lb sautéed fresh or frozen snap peas

Tossed Garden Salad (page 211)

DESSERT FOR 4 (OPTIONAL)

Caramelized Pineapple Rings (page 234)

OR

WLE 2 fresh or canned unsweetened pineapple rings per person

Daily Nutrition Facts

REGULAR

1,459 calories: 19% from fat (5% from sat fat), 20% from protein, 62% from carbohydrate; 33 g fiber, 176 mg cholesterol, 1,392 mg sodium

WEIGHT-LOSS EXPRESS

1,281 calories: 18% from fat (3% from sat fat), 20% from protein, 62% from carbohydrate; 25 g fiber, 175 mg cholesterol, 1,142 mg sodium

DAY 3 **CRANBERRY DAY**

BREAKFAST

2 Cranberry-Banana Soft Wheat Muffins (page 143)

1 cup fat-free milk

OR

WLE Cranberry-Banana Smoothie (page 150)

MIDMORNING SNACK

$^{1}/_{2}$ cup fat-free plain yogurt with 2 tsp dried cranberries and 1 Tbsp low-fat granola

LUNCH

Cranberry-Lentil Mixed Greens Salad with Feta and Pecans (page 168)

MIDAFTERNOON SNACK

Cranberry-Banana Smoothie (page 150)

DINNER FOR 4

Cranberry and Sweet Onion Turkey Cutlets (page 197)

Baked sweet potatoes (wrap 2 whole sweet potatoes in aluminum foil and bake at 375°F until tender; unwrap and cut each in half for 1 serving)

Tossed Garden Salad (page 211; add 2 tsp dried cranberries)

DESSERT FOR 4 (OPTIONAL)

Cranberry-Vanilla Soft Ice Cream (page 243)

OR

WLE No dessert

Daily Nutrition Facts

REGULAR

1,453 calories: 20% from fat (3% from sat fat), 23% from protein, 57% from carbohydrate; 24 g fiber, 150 mg cholesterol, 1,272 mg sodium

WEIGHT-LOSS EXPRESS

1,272 calories: 17% from fat (3% from sat fat), 23% from protein, 60% from carbohydrate; 24 g fiber, 117 mg cholesterol, 1,062 mg sodium

DAY 4 **LEMON DAY**

BREAKFAST

2 Lemon-Poppy Soft Wheat Muffins (page 145)

OR

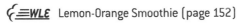 Lemon-Orange Smoothie (page 152)

MIDMORNING SNACK

³/₄ cup fat-free lemon yogurt with ¹/₄ cup whole grain cereal

LUNCH

Lemon Tabbouleh Salad (page 167)

MIDAFTERNOON SNACK

Lemon-Orange Smoothie (page 152)

OR

 ¹/₂ cup fat-free cottage cheese

12 oz lemon fizz (10 oz seltzer water and juice of ¹/₂ lemon)

DINNER FOR 4

Pan-Seared Tilapia with Lemon Chives and Capers (page 203)

1 lb sautéed fresh or frozen asparagus with grated lemon peel

Baked fries (bake 1 bag Alexia julienne fries according to package directions)

Tossed Garden Salad (page 211; add juice of ¹/₂ lemon)

DESSERT FOR 4 (OPTIONAL)

4 cups fresh blueberries with lemon peel; 1 cup per person

Daily Nutrition Facts

REGULAR

1,415 calories: 23% from fat (3% from sat fat), 19% from protein, 57% from carbohydrate; 30 g fiber, 150 mg cholesterol, 1,281 mg sodium

WEIGHT-LOSS EXPRESS

1,257 calories: 20% from fat (3% from sat fat), 23% from protein, 57% from carbohydrate; 27 g fiber, 94 mg cholesterol, 1,551 mg sodium

DAY 5 **PEACH DAY**

BREAKFAST

1 cup whole grain cereal with ½ cup fat-free milk

1 fresh peach or ½ cup canned unsweetened peaches

MIDMORNING SNACK

½ cup fat-free peach yogurt with 1 Tbsp chopped pecans

LUNCH

Peanut butter and peach jam sandwich (2 slices whole grain bread, 1 Tbsp natural peanut butter, and 1 Tbsp all-fruit peach jam)

1 cup fat-free milk

OR

 Peach-Banana Smoothie (page 151)

MIDAFTERNOON SNACK

½ cup canned unsweetened peaches

DINNER FOR 4

Peach-Coriander Turkey with Oven-Roasted Potatoes and Turnips (page 198)

Tossed Garden Salad (page 211)

DESSERT FOR 6 (OPTIONAL)

Peach Flat Cake (page 235)

OR

 1 ripe peach per person

Daily Nutrition Facts

REGULAR

1,493 calories: 23% from fat (4% from sat fat), 19% from protein, 57% from carbohydrate; 37 g fiber, 160 mg cholesterol, 1,825 mg sodium

WEIGHT-LOSS EXPRESS

1,204 calories: 17% from fat (3% from sat fat), 18% from protein, 64% from carbohydrate; 31 g fiber, 97 mg cholesterol, 1,438 mg sodium

DAY 6 **ORANGE DAY**

BREAKFAST

1 cup whole grain cereal with $\frac{1}{2}$ cup fat-free milk

$\frac{3}{4}$ cup 100% orange juice

OR

WLE Orange-Banana Smoothie (page 151)

MIDMORNING SNACK

$\frac{1}{2}$ cup fat-free plain yogurt with 1 sliced orange and 2 tsp raisins

OR

WLE Omit the yogurt and raisins

LUNCH

Orange-Lentil Spinach Salad with Feta and Pecans (page 169)

MIDAFTERNOON SNACK

Orange-Banana Smoothie (page 151)

OR

WLE 10 oz orange fizz (6 oz seltzer water and 4 oz 100% orange juice)

DINNER FOR 4

CN Orange Grilled Tuna (page 205)

4 cups cooked bulgur wheat (page 228)

1 lb sautéed fresh or frozen French-cut string beans with grated orange peel

Tossed Garden Salad (page 211; add juice of $\frac{1}{2}$ orange)

DESSERT FOR 4 (OPTIONAL)

Fat-free orange sorbet; $\frac{1}{2}$ cup per person

OR

WLE 1 sliced orange per person

Daily Nutrition Facts

REGULAR

1,499 calories: 18% from fat (3% from sat fat), 20% from protein, 62% from carbohydrate; 38 g fiber, 83 mg cholesterol, 1,248 mg sodium

WEIGHT-LOSS EXPRESS

1,214 calories: 22% from fat (3% from sat fat), 21% from protein, 58% from carbohydrate; 34 g fiber, 79 mg cholesterol, 928 mg sodium

DAY 7 **APPLE DAY**

BREAKFAST

Apple-Raisin Oatmeal (page 141)

OR

WLE Apple-Banana Smoothie (page 150)

MIDMORNING SNACK

$1/2$ cup unsweetened applesauce

$1/2$ cup fat-free plain yogurt

LUNCH

Apple-Walnut Chicken Salad (page 176)

5 Kashi TLC Original 7-Grain Crackers

MIDAFTERNOON SNACK

$1/2$ sliced apple spread with 1 Tbsp natural peanut butter

OR

WLE 10 oz apple fizz (6 oz seltzer water and 4 oz 100% apple juice)

DINNER FOR 4

Apple–Butternut Squash Soup (page 217)

2 slices whole grain bread per person

Tossed Garden Salad (page 211)

DESSERT FOR 4 (OPTIONAL)

Warm Apple Crisp (page 242)

Daily Nutrition Facts

REGULAR

1,424 calories: 22% from fat (3% from sat fat), 18% from protein, 60% from carbohydrate; 40 g fiber, 76 mg cholesterol, 1,361 mg sodium

WEIGHT-LOSS EXPRESS

1,236 calories: 18% from fat (3% from sat fat), 17% from protein, 65% from carbohydrate; 33 g fiber, 75 mg cholesterol, 1,313 mg sodium

WEEK 2

DAY 8 **TOMATO DAY**

DAY 9 **CARROT DAY**

DAY 10 **MUSHROOM DAY**

DAY 11 **ONION DAY**

DAY 12 **PUMPKIN DAY** **CN**

DAY 13 **SPINACH DAY**

DAY 14 **BELL PEPPER DAY**

DAY 8 **TOMATO DAY**

BREAKFAST

Tomato and egg sandwich (2 slices whole grain bread, 1 soft-cooked egg, 2 slices tomato, and 1 Tbsp grated part-skim mozzarella, melted)

OR

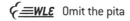 Use 1 slice bread and omit the cheese and 1 slice tomato

MIDMORNING SNACK

12 cherry tomatoes with 2 Tbsp hummus

OR

≡WLE Omit the hummus

LUNCH

Tomato and Black Bean Mediterranean Salad (page 173) in ½ whole wheat pita

OR

≡WLE Omit the pita

MIDAFTERNOON SNACK

12 baked corn chips with ⅓ cup tomato salsa

OR

≡WLE Replace the chips with 12 baby carrots

DINNER FOR 4

Baked Tilapia with Tomatoes, Olives, and Capers (page 202)

4 cups cooked bulgur wheat (page 228)

12 oz sautéed fresh or frozen cauliflower florets

Tossed Garden Salad (page 211; add 1½ cups rinsed and drained chickpeas)

DESSERT FOR 4 (OPTIONAL)

Peach-blueberry salad (2 cups fresh or canned peach slices and 2 cups blueberries); 1 cup per person

---

Daily Nutrition Facts

REGULAR

1,535 calories: 24% from fat (5% from sat fat), 20% from protein, 56% from carbohydrate; 53 g fiber, 272 mg cholesterol, 2,186 mg sodium

WEIGHT-LOSS EXPRESS

1,289 calories: 27% from fat (5% from sat fat), 22% from protein, 52% from carbohydrate; 44 g fiber, 270 mg cholesterol, 1,884 mg sodium

DAY 9 **CARROT DAY**

BREAKFAST

1 cup whole grain cereal with ½ cup fat-free milk

¾ cup 100% carrot-orange juice

OR

WLE Carrot-Pineapple Smoothie (page 150)

MIDMORNING SNACK

Up to 18 baby carrots with ½ cup fat-free cottage cheese

LUNCH

Carrot, hummus, tomato, and avocado sandwich (2 slices whole grain bread, 2 Tbsp hummus, ½ cup grated carrots, ¼ sliced avocado, ½ sliced tomato, and alfalfa sprouts to taste)

OR

WLE Omit the avocado

MIDAFTERNOON SNACK

Up to 18 baby carrots with ⅓ cup fat-free bean dip

OR

WLE Omit the bean dip

DINNER FOR 4

Carrot Cider–Glazed Chicken (page 180)

3 cups cooked brown rice (page 228)

1 lb sautéed fresh or frozen broccoli rabe

Tossed Garden Salad (page 211)

DESSERT FOR 4 (OPTIONAL)

Oranges with honey yogurt drizzle (peel and slice 4 oranges; whisk together ½ cup fat-free plain yogurt and 1 Tbsp honey); 1 cup per person

---

Daily Nutrition Facts

REGULAR

1,515 calories: 19% from fat (3% from sat fat), 21% from protein, 60% from carbohydrate; 41 g fiber, 97 mg cholesterol, 2,115 mg sodium

WEIGHT-LOSS EXPRESS

1,244 calories: 17% from fat (3% from sat fat), 21% from protein, 62% from carbohydrate; 29 g fiber, 96 mg cholesterol, 1,591 mg sodium

DAY 10 **MUSHROOM DAY**

BREAKFAST

Mushroom, Thyme, and Cheese Omelet (page 149)

1 slice whole grain toast, plain or with 1 tsp Smart Balance spread

MIDMORNING SNACK

10 baby carrots with Mushroom Dip (page 156)

OR

 2 sliced celery stalks with Mushroom Dip

LUNCH

Portobello Mushroom, Gorgonzola, and Sun-Dried Tomato Sandwich (page 175)

OR

 Omit the gorgonzola

MIDAFTERNOON SNACK

10 Kashi TLC Original 7-Grain Crackers with Mushroom Dip (page 156)

OR

 10 bell pepper strips with Mushroom Dip

DINNER FOR 4

Chicken in Creamy Dijon Mushroom Sauce (page 184)

3 cups cooked brown rice (page 228)

1 lb sautéed fresh or frozen broccoli florets

Tossed Garden Salad (page 211; add fresh mushrooms)

DESSERT FOR 4 (OPTIONAL)

Fruit salad (1 sliced banana; 2 medium apples, cored and cut into small chunks; and 24 grapes); $^3/_4$ cup per person

---

Daily Nutrition Facts

REGULAR

1,469 calories: 22% from fat (5% from sat fat), 25% from protein, 52% from carbohydrate; 38 g fiber, 454 mg cholesterol, 2,013 mg sodium

WEIGHT-LOSS EXPRESS

1,347 calories: 21% from fat (5% from sat fat), 26% from protein, 51% from carbohydrate; 37 g fiber, 448 mg cholesterol, 1,851 mg sodium

DAY 11 **ONION DAY**

BREAKFAST

Green Scallion and Cheese Omelet (page 149)

1 slice whole grain toast, plain or with 1 tsp Smart Balance spread

MIDMORNING SNACK

10 baby carrots and celery sticks with Scallion Yogurt Dip (page 157)

LUNCH

Red Onion, White Bean, Lentil, and Tomato Salad (page 171)

4 Stacy's Simply Naked Baked Pita Chips

OR

≡WLE Omit the beans and chips and add 1 tomato

MIDAFTERNOON SNACK

10 Kashi TLC Original 7-Grain Crackers with Scallion Yogurt Dip (page 157)

OR

≡WLE Replace the crackers with 1 cucumber cut into sticks

DINNER FOR 4

Grilled Chicken with Caramelized Onion on Pita (page 189)

Cucumber, Tomato, Olive, and Red Onion Salad (page 212)

DESSERT FOR 4 (OPTIONAL)

Fruit salad (1 sliced banana; 2 medium apples, cored and cut into small chunks; and 24 grapes); ³⁄₄ cup per person

Daily Nutrition Facts

REGULAR

1,436 calories: 31% from fat (6% from sat fat), 21% from protein, 48% from carbohydrate; 35 g fiber, 445 mg cholesterol, 2,127 mg sodium

WEIGHT-LOSS EXPRESS

1,298 calories: 32% from fat (6% from sat fat), 22% from protein, 46% from carbohydrate; 33 g fiber, 445 mg cholesterol, 1,749 mg sodium

Satisfaction at the Flavor Point

THE FLAVOR FACTS

Name: Carol Borger

Age: 46

Hometown: Hamden, Connecticut

Family status: Married with two children, ages 15 and 17

Occupation: Phlebotomist

Starting weight: 183

Pounds lost: 17 in 12 weeks

Health stats: Blood pressure dropped 15 points; cholesterol dropped 54 points; irritable bowel flare-ups have disappeared; 5½ percent decline in body fat

---

"Until recently, I only knew how to cook meat and potatoes. That's what my mother cooked, so that's what I cooked. When I found out that my cholesterol was 300, and my husband's and two kids' levels were all over 200, I said, 'That's it—we have to do something.' When I heard about Dr. Katz's program, I knew I had found that something.

"For the most part, my family has been on board because they know I'm doing this for the right reasons.

They liked the food I used to cook, but they're learning to accept the fact that it was horrible for us and that we all needed to make a change. I can't say they've been as strict as I have, but they've been doing most of the program with me. My husband has lost 21 pounds so far.

"I've been choosing flavor-friendly options for breakfast and lunch, but when it comes time for dinner, I'm amazed at how easy it is to cook healthfully. I made peanut butter shrimp the other night, and other than peeling the shrimp, it was simple, and it tasted absolutely amazing. The coconut chicken has also been a big hit, along with the stuffed peppers with bulgur wheat and ground turkey and the tilapia with lemon sauce. I've also started improvising with some of the recipes. I created breading with flour and Kashi crackers and made great breaded haddock and chicken Parmesan with it.

"All the flavors on the program help make it more interesting and satisfying, and the themes have introduced me to new foods and spices. I've also learned some great tricks for saving calories, like using plain yogurt instead of mayo in chicken salad and ground turkey instead of ground beef. I slipped some ground turkey into a recipe and told my husband it was beef—he had no idea! And my kitchen is stocked with new brands, like Alexia fries and Kashi crackers. Now, when my kids come home from school, they munch on high-fiber cereal instead of chips. We've also been making a lot of the smoothies with fresh fruit and vanilla yogurt. The blender gets a lot of use in our house!

"I'm totally satisfied on the plan. There is more food on our table than ever before, but fewer calories. If I do start to feel a little hungry, I reach for a piece of fruit. It's amazing. I don't miss the red meat at all. I haven't craved red meat since I started. I also don't crave sweets like I used to. My son just headed out the door to go to Dairy Queen, and I wasn't the least bit tempted to ask him to pick something up for me.

"Health-wise, the program has done wonders for me. Not only have I lost 20 pounds, but my cholesterol and triglycerides dropped, and I lost more than 4 inches off my waist. Before I started, I had regular symptoms of irritable bowel syndrome, and they've completely disappeared. The other night, I had a piece of pizza and felt uncomfortable and bloated for 2 days. It reminded me of how bad my old eating habits used to make me feel.

"I also love the way I look. The other day, I was shopping for new clothes with my daughter, and I caught a glimpse of myself in a mirror. I backed up to take a second look and said, 'Wow!' I'm 46 years old, I just lost 17 pounds, and I'm fitting into a size 10. I'm pretty happy with that! And everybody notices the change, especially in my face. I've lost a few chins, and my butt looks cute now.

"This program has truly changed my life. It's so rewarding to see my cholesterol and triglycerides go down without medication. I know I can stick with this. I've made the change, and this is the way I and my whole family are going to eat from now on." ■

DAY 12 **PUMPKIN DAY**

BREAKFAST

2 Pumpkin-Banana Soft Wheat Muffins (page 144)

OR

 1 slice whole grain toast with 1 Tbsp pumpkin butter and 2 tsp natural peanut butter

MIDMORNING SNACK

Pumpkin-Allspice Smoothie (page 152)

LUNCH

Pumpkin and Chocolate Grilled Panini (page 178)

¾ cup fat-free milk

MIDAFTERNOON SNACK

Pumpkin-Allspice Smoothie (page 152)

DINNER FOR 4

 Pumpkin Soup (page 223)

2 slices whole grain bread per person

OR

 Omit 1 slice bread per person

Tossed Garden Salad (page 211; add 1½ cups rinsed and drained chickpeas and 2 oz feta)

DESSERT FOR 4 (OPTIONAL)

Pumpkin Soft Ice Cream (page 244)

Daily Nutrition Facts

REGULAR

1,461 calories: 22% from fat (4% from sat fat), 18% from protein, 61% from carbohydrate; 50 g fiber, 67 mg cholesterol, 1,855 mg sodium

WEIGHT-LOSS EXPRESS

1,290 calories: 19% from fat (4% from sat fat), 18% from protein, 63% from carbohydrate; 47 g fiber, 6 mg cholesterol, 1,762 mg sodium

DAY 13 **SPINACH DAY**

BREAKFAST

Spinach and Feta Omelet (page 149)

1 slice whole grain toast, plain or with 1 tsp Smart Balance spread

OR

 ¾ cup whole grain cereal with ½ cup fat-free milk

MIDMORNING SNACK

10 Kashi TLC Original 7-Grain Crackers with Spinach Yogurt Dip (page 158)

LUNCH

Spinach and Turkey Chef's Salad (page 172)

MIDAFTERNOON SNACK

Up to 18 baby carrots with Spinach Yogurt Dip (page 158)

DINNER FOR 4

Pasta Fagioli with Spinach Marinara Sauce (page 215)

Tossed Garden Salad (page 211; make with spinach)

DESSERT FOR 4 (OPTIONAL)

Mixed-berry salad (1 cup each fresh blueberries, raspberries, and black-
berries); ¾ cup per person

OR

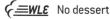 No dessert

---

Daily Nutrition Facts

REGULAR

1,449 calories: 27% from fat (5% from sat
fat), 20% from protein, 54% from carbohydrate; 47 g fiber, 408 mg cholesterol, 2,715
mg sodium

WEIGHT-LOSS EXPRESS

1,284 calories: 21% from fat (3% from sat
fat), 19% from protein, 59% from carbohydrate; 43 g fiber, 44 mg cholesterol, 2,284
mg sodium

DAY 14 **BELL PEPPER DAY**

BREAKFAST

Bell Pepper and Cheese Omelet (page 148)

1 slice whole grain toast, plain or with 1 tsp Smart Balance spread

OR

$\langle \equiv$**WLE** $^{3}/_{4}$ cup whole grain cereal with $^{1}/_{2}$ cup fat-free milk

MIDMORNING SNACK

Up to 18 baby carrots with Bell Pepper Yogurt Dip (page 155)

LUNCH

Roasted pepper, avocado, and hummus sandwich (2 slices whole grain bread, 2 oz roasted bell peppers, 3 Tbsp hummus, $^{1}/_{4}$ ripe black avocado, and alfalfa sprouts to taste)

MIDAFTERNOON SNACK

2 Wasa Rye Crispbreads with Bell Pepper Yogurt Dip (page 155)

DINNER FOR 4

Mexican Stuffed Bell Peppers (page 193)

1 lb sautéed frozen whole-kernel sweet corn

Tossed Garden Salad (page 211; add $^{1}/_{2}$ cup chopped bell pepper)

DESSERT FOR 4 (OPTIONAL)

Fruit salad (2 cups cubed cantaloupe, 2 cups cubed honeydew, and $1^{1}/_{2}$ cups fresh or frozen raspberries); $1^{1}/_{3}$ cups per person

Daily Nutrition Facts

REGULAR

1,427 calories: 25% from fat (6% from sat fat), 17% from protein, 58% from carbohydrate; 50 g fiber, 420 mg cholesterol, 2,340 mg sodium

WEIGHT-LOSS EXPRESS

1,246 calories: 22% from fat (4% from sat fat), 17% from protein, 62% from carbohydrate; 47 g fiber, 59 mg cholesterol, 1,870 mg sodium

WEEK 3

DAY 15 **APPLE DAY**

DAY 16 **TOMATO DAY**   CN)

DAY 17 **ALMOND DAY**

DAY 18 **THYME DAY**

DAY 19 **WALNUT DAY**

DAY 20 **SESAME DAY**   CN)

DAY 21 **BASIL DAY**

DAY 15 **APPLE DAY**

BREAKFAST

Apple Multigrain Pancakes with Honey Yogurt Sauce (page 146)

OR

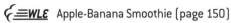 Apple-Banana Smoothie (page 150)

MIDMORNING SNACK

$\frac{1}{2}$ cup unsweetened applesauce mixed with $\frac{1}{2}$ cup fat-free plain yogurt

OR

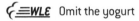 Omit the yogurt

LUNCH

Apple, Fennel, Walnut, and Barley Salad (page 163)

MIDAFTERNOON SNACK

1 small apple

OR

≡WLE 10 oz apple fizz (6 oz seltzer water and 4 oz 100% apple juice)

DINNER FOR 4

Apple-Prune Chicken (page 196)

4 cups cooked bulgur wheat (page 228)

12 oz sautéed spinach

Tossed Garden Salad (page 211)

DESSERT FOR 4 (OPTIONAL)

Baked Cinnamon Apples (page 231)

Daily Nutrition Facts

REGULAR

1,459 calories: 19% from fat (3% from sat fat), 17% from protein, 64% from carbohydrate; 48 g fiber, 125 mg cholesterol, 1,697 mg sodium

WEIGHT-LOSS EXPRESS

1,285 calories: 18% from fat (3% from sat fat), 15% from protein, 67% from carbohydrate; 41 g fiber, 76 mg cholesterol, 1,329 mg sodium

DAY 16 **TOMATO DAY**

BREAKFAST

Tomato, Basil, and Feta Omelet (page 149)

1 slice whole grain toast, plain or with 1 tsp Smart Balance spread

OR

 1 slice whole grain bread, 1 thick slice tomato, and ½ Tbsp grated part-skim mozzarella, melted

MIDMORNING SNACK

12 cherry tomatoes with 2 Tbsp hummus

OR

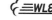 Omit the hummus

LUNCH

Tomato and Black Bean Mediterranean Salad (page 173) in ½ whole wheat pita

MIDAFTERNOON SNACK

12 baked corn chips with ⅓ cup tomato salsa

OR

 Replace the chips with 12 baby carrots

DINNER FOR 4

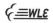 Pasta with Marinara Sauce (page 216)

Tossed Garden Salad (page 211; add 2 cups rinsed and drained chickpeas)

Whole Wheat Garlic Bread (page 227)

DESSERT FOR 4 (OPTIONAL)

Peach-blueberry salad (2 cups fresh or canned peach slices and 2 cups blueberries); 1 cup per person

OR

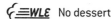 No dessert

---

Daily Nutrition Facts

REGULAR

1,508 calories: 25% from fat (5% from sat fat), 15% from protein, 60% from carbohydrate; 53 g fiber, 370 mg cholesterol, 1,889 mg sodium

WEIGHT-LOSS EXPRESS

1,307 calories: 23% from fat (5% from sat fat), 15% from protein, 63% from carbohydrate; 51 g fiber, 190 mg cholesterol, 1,430 mg sodium

DAY 17 **ALMOND DAY**

BREAKFAST

2 slices Almond French Toast with Sliced Strawberries (page 140)

MIDMORNING SNACK

Almond-Banana Smoothie (page 150)

OR

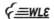 ½ cup fat-free plain yogurt with 6 whole almonds

LUNCH

Almond, Green Bean, and Quinoa Salad (page 162)

MIDAFTERNOON SNACK

10–12 whole almonds and 1 fresh pear or ½ cup canned unsweetened pears

OR

 6 whole almonds and 1 Tbsp raisins

DINNER FOR 4

Almond-Crusted Tilapia (page 201)

1 lb sautéed fresh or frozen broccoli florets with 1 Tbsp sliced almonds

Tossed Garden Salad (page 211)

DESSERT FOR 4 (OPTIONAL)

Amaretto strawberry salad (3 cups sliced strawberries, 4 tsp amaretto liqueur, and 4 tsp chopped almonds); ¾ cup per person

---

Daily Nutrition Facts

REGULAR

1,479 calories: 36% from fat (5% from sat fat), 21% from protein, 42% from carbohydrate; 43 g fiber, 266 mg cholesterol, 1,272 mg sodium

WEIGHT-LOSS EXPRESS

1,309 calories: 39% from fat (6% from sat fat), 22% from protein, 39% from carbohydrate; 38 g fiber, 267 mg cholesterol, 1,226 mg sodium

DAY 18 **THYME DAY**

BREAKFAST

Mushroom, Thyme, and Cheese Omelet (page 149)

1 slice whole grain toast, plain or with 1 tsp Smart Balance spread

OR

 Scrambled Eggs with Thyme (page 147)

1 slice whole grain toast, plain or with 1 tsp Smart Balance spread

MIDMORNING SNACK

Up to 18 baby carrots with Thyme Yogurt Dip (page 159)

LUNCH

Stuffed Tomato with Thyme Tuna Salad (page 174)

5 Kashi TLC Original 7-Grain Crackers

OR

 Omit the crackers

MIDAFTERNOON SNACK

6 Snyder's of Hanover Oat Bran Sticks

$\frac{1}{4}$ cup fat-free cottage cheese with $\frac{1}{4}$ tsp dried or 1 tsp fresh thyme

DINNER FOR 4

Grilled Chicken with White Beans Provençal (page 190)

4 cups cooked bulgur wheat (page 228)

Tossed Garden Salad (page 211)

DESSERT FOR 4 (OPTIONAL)

Fruit salad (1 sliced banana; 2 medium apples, cored and cut into small chunks; and 24 grapes); $\frac{3}{4}$ cup per person

---

Daily Nutrition Facts

REGULAR

1,422 calories: 22% from fat (5% from sat fat), 26% from protein, 50% from carbohydrate; 41 g fiber, 455 mg cholesterol, 2,472 mg sodium

WEIGHT-LOSS EXPRESS

1,255 calories: 20% from fat (4% from sat fat), 28% from protein, 49% from carbohydrate; 34 g fiber, 450 mg cholesterol, 2,287 mg sodium

DAY 19 **WALNUT DAY**

BREAKFAST

Walnut Multigrain Pancakes with Honey Yogurt Sauce (page 147)

OR

WLE ³/₄ cup fat-free plain yogurt with ¹/₄ cup low-fat walnut granola

MIDMORNING SNACK

¹/₂ cup fat-free plain yogurt with 1 Tbsp chopped walnuts and 1 Tbsp raisins

OR

WLE 1 Tbsp chopped walnuts and 1 dried apricot

LUNCH

Walnut Chicken Salad (page 176)

5 Stacy's Simply Naked Baked Pita Chips

OR

WLE Omit the chips

MIDAFTERNOON SNACK

6 walnut halves and 16 grapes

OR

WLE Omit the grapes

DINNER FOR 4

Portobello Mushrooms with Walnut Stuffing (page 220)

12 oz baby spinach sautéed in 1 tsp olive oil with 1 Tbsp chopped walnuts

Lentil and Bean Salad with Cilantro (page 213) over mixed greens

DESSERT FOR 4 (OPTIONAL)

Baked Cinnamon-Walnut Apples (page 231)

Daily Nutrition Facts

REGULAR

1,526 calories: 35% from fat (5% from sat fat), 20% from protein, 46% from carbohydrate; 32 g fiber, 128 mg cholesterol, 1,459 mg sodium

WEIGHT-LOSS EXPRESS

1,289 calories: 36% from fat (5% from sat fat), 21% from protein, 43% from carbohydrate; 28 g fiber, 83 mg cholesterol, 1,139 mg sodium

DAY 20 **SESAME DAY**

BREAKFAST

2 slices Sesame French Toast with Sliced Strawberries (page 141)

MIDMORNING SNACK

1 cup chopped fresh vegetables (8 baby carrots and celery sticks) with Tahini Dip (page 157)

LUNCH

Carrot, hummus, lettuce, and tomato sandwich (2 slices whole grain bread, 2 Tbsp hummus, ½ cup grated carrots, ½ sliced tomato, and lettuce)

MIDAFTERNOON SNACK

2 Ak-Mak 100% Whole Wheat Sesame Crackers with Tahini Dip (page 157)

OR

 Replace the crackers with 10 celery sticks

DINNER FOR 4

CN Sesame-Soy Chicken Cutlets (page 179)

1 lb sautéed bean sprouts

Tossed Garden Salad (page 211)

DESSERT FOR 4 (OPTIONAL)

4 sliced fresh pears or 1½ cups canned pear slices sprinkled with ¼ cup sesame seeds; 1 fresh pear or about ⅔ cup canned pears per person

OR

 No dessert

Daily Nutrition Facts

REGULAR

1,471 calories: 30% from fat (5% from sat fat), 19% from protein, 50% from carbohydrate; 46 g fiber, 274 mg cholesterol, 1,802 mg sodium

WEIGHT-LOSS EXPRESS

1,291 calories: 31% from fat (6% from sat fat), 21% from protein, 47% from carbohydrate; 42 g fiber, 274 mg cholesterol, 1,901 mg sodium

DAY 21 **BASIL DAY**

BREAKFAST

Tomato, Basil, and Feta Omelet (page 149)

1 slice whole grain toast, plain or with 1 tsp Smart Balance spread

OR

 1 slice whole wheat bread with ½ chopped tomato, 5 chopped fresh basil leaves, and 1 Tbsp grated part-skim mozzarella, melted

MIDMORNING SNACK

10 green beans, 6 baby carrots, and 6 cauliflower florets with Basil-Ricotta Dip (page 154)

LUNCH

Turkey sandwich with basil, lettuce, and tomato (2 slices whole grain bread, 2 slices unprocessed roast turkey, 2 tsp pesto basil spread, lettuce, and ½ sliced tomato)

MIDAFTERNOON SNACK

6 Snyder's of Hanover Oat Bran Sticks with 2 Tbsp hummus mixed with 5 chopped fresh basil leaves

OR

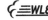 Replace the oat bran sticks with 10 celery sticks

DINNER FOR 4

Shrimp Pasta Primavera with Basil Pesto (page 209)

Tossed Garden Salad (page 211; add fresh basil to taste)

DESSERT FOR 4 (OPTIONAL)

Strawberry-kiwi salad (2 cups sliced strawberries and 3 sliced kiwis); ¾ cup per person

---

Daily Nutrition Facts

REGULAR

1,490 calories: 34% from fat (6% from sat fat), 21% from protein, 45% from carbohydrate; 46 g fiber, 494 mg cholesterol, 2,232 mg sodium

WEIGHT-LOSS EXPRESS

1,297 calories: 31% from fat (5% from sat fat), 20% from protein, 50% from carbohydrate; 47 g fiber, 135 mg cholesterol, 1,734 mg sodium

WEEK 4

DAY 22 **SPINACH DAY**

DAY 23 **ORANGE DAY**   CN

DAY 24 **MINT DAY**

DAY 25 **LEMON DAY**

DAY 26 **PECAN DAY**

DAY 27 **DILL DAY**

DAY 28 **CRANBERRY DAY**

DAY 22 **SPINACH DAY**

BREAKFAST

Spinach and Feta Omelet (page 149)

1 slice whole grain toast, plain or with 1 tsp Smart Balance spread

OR

 ¾ cup whole grain cereal with ½ cup fat-free milk

MIDMORNING SNACK

10 Kashi TLC Original 7-Grain Crackers with Spinach Yogurt Dip (page 158)

LUNCH

Spinach and Turkey Chef's Salad (page 172)

MIDAFTERNOON SNACK

12 baby carrots with Spinach Yogurt Dip (page 158)

DINNER FOR 4

Pasta Fagioli with Spinach Marinara Sauce (page 215)

Tossed Garden Salad (page 211; make with spinach)

DESSERT FOR 4 (OPTIONAL)

Mixed-berry salad (1 cup each fresh blueberries, raspberries, and black-berries); ¾ cup per person

OR

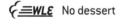 No dessert

---

Daily Nutrition Facts

REGULAR

1,449 calories: 27% from fat (5% from sat fat), 20% from protein, 54% from carbohydrate; 47 g fiber, 408 mg cholesterol, 2,715 mg sodium

WEIGHT-LOSS EXPRESS

1,284 calories: 21% from fat (3% from sat fat), 19% from protein, 59% from carbohydrate; 43 g fiber, 44 mg cholesterol, 2,284 mg sodium

DAY 23 **ORANGE DAY**

BREAKFAST

1 cup whole grain cereal with ¹/₂ cup fat-free milk

³/₄ cup 100% orange juice

OR

WLE Orange-Banana Smoothie (page 151)

MIDMORNING SNACK

¹/₂ cup fat-free plain yogurt with 1 sliced orange

LUNCH

Orange-Lentil Spinach Salad with Feta and Pecans (page 169)

MIDAFTERNOON SNACK

Orange-Banana Smoothie (page 151)

OR

WLE 10 oz orange fizz (6 oz seltzer water and 4 oz 100% orange juice)

DINNER FOR 4

 Orange Cod (page 204)

1 lb sautéed fresh or frozen French-cut string beans with grated orange peel

4 cups cooked bulgur wheat (page 228)

Tossed Garden Salad (page 211; add juice of ¹/₂ orange)

DESSERT FOR 4 (OPTIONAL)

Fat-free orange sorbet; ¹/₂ cup per person

OR

WLE 1 orange

Daily Nutrition Facts

REGULAR

1,431 calories: 20% from fat (3% from sat fat), 16% from protein, 64% from carbohydrate; 39 g fiber, 35 mg cholesterol, 1,509 mg sodium

WEIGHT-LOSS EXPRESS

1,196 calories: 23% from fat (3% from sat fat), 17% from protein, 61% from carbohydrate; 34 g fiber, 33 mg cholesterol, 1,256 mg sodium

DAY 24 **MINT DAY**

BREAKFAST

1½ cups whole grain cereal with ¾ cup milk

1 cup peppermint tea with 1 tsp honey

MIDMORNING SNACK

1 cup sliced fresh strawberries sprinkled with chopped fresh mint

1 cup peppermint tea with 1 tsp honey

LUNCH

Fresh Mint Salade Niçoise (page 166)

MIDAFTERNOON SNACK

1 banana

1 cup peppermint tea with 1 tsp honey

DINNER FOR 4

Mint, Sweet Pea, and Spinach Soup (page 222)

1 slice whole grain bread per person

Minty Tabbouleh Salad (page 214)

OR

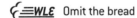 Omit the bread

DESSERT FOR 4 (OPTIONAL)

Mint Chocolate Chip Shake (page 243)

OR

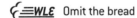 No dessert

---

Daily Nutrition Facts

REGULAR

1,498 calories: 19% from fat (3% from sat fat), 20% from protein, 61% from carbohydrate; 52 g fiber, 204 mg cholesterol, 2,423 mg sodium

WEIGHT-LOSS EXPRESS

1,319 calories: 21% from fat (4% from sat fat), 21% from protein, 59% from carbohydrate; 46 g fiber, 201 mg cholesterol, 2,258 mg sodium

DAY 25 **LEMON DAY**

BREAKFAST

2 Lemon-Poppy Soft Wheat Muffins (page 145)

OR

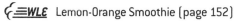 Lemon-Orange Smoothie (page 152)

MIDMORNING SNACK

³/₄ cup fat-free lemon yogurt with ¹/₄ cup whole grain cereal

LUNCH

Lemon Tabbouleh Salad (page 167)

MIDAFTERNOON SNACK

Lemon-Orange Smoothie (page 152)

OR

 ¹/₂ cup fat-free cottage cheese and 12 oz lemon fizz (10 oz seltzer water and juice of ¹/₂ lemon)

DINNER FOR 4

Lemon Salmon with Garlic Spinach (page 206)

Sautéed Spaghetti Squash (page 225)

1 slice whole grain bread per person

Tossed Garden Salad (page 211; add juice of ¹/₂ lemon)

OR

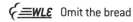 Omit the bread

DESSERT FOR 4 (OPTIONAL)

4 cups fresh blueberries with lemon peel; 1 cup per person

Daily Nutrition Facts

REGULAR

1,456 calories: 24% from fat (3% from sat fat), 20% from protein, 56% from carbohydrate; 36 g fiber, 175 mg cholesterol, 1,532 mg sodium

WEIGHT-LOSS EXPRESS

1,238 calories: 21% from fat (3% from sat fat), 25% from protein, 54% from carbohydrate; 29 g fiber, 118 mg cholesterol, 1,722 mg sodium

Satisfaction at the Flavor Point

THE FLAVOR FACTS

Name: Cindy Garafolo

Age: 46

Hometown: Beacon Falls, Connecticut

Family status: Married with two children, ages 19 and 20

Occupation: Medical assistant

Starting weight: 173

Pounds lost: 13½ in 12 weeks

Health stats: Cholesterol dropped 18 points; blood pressure dropped 8 points; waist measurement shrank 2½ inches; 5 percent decline in body fat

"My husband and I both wanted to lose weight, so Dr. Katz's program just came up at the right time. I had no idea what I was getting into, but it has really worked! My husband and I both lost about 14 pounds in the first 12 weeks.

"Before I started the program, I would eat more out of boredom than hunger. I didn't even think about it. Dr. Katz has taught me to be more conscious of whether or not I'm really hungry. If I think I'm genuinely hungry, I now grab a piece of fruit or one of the snacks, like a fruit-and-yogurt parfait or a smoothie rather than candy.

"For breakfast, I usually choose one of the flavor-friendly options, like oatmeal. For lunch, my whole family's favorite is the chicken salad with yogurt and mustard. My daughter asks me to make it for her all the time. For dinner, I love the chicken recipes, especially Roast Chicken with Currant Wine Glaze and Caramelized Onions. The currants cook down and make the sauce thick, like gravy. This recipe would be great for a party.

"Overall, my food preferences have absolutely changed on Dr. Katz's program. This meal plan has turned my entire family on to foods we wouldn't have tried otherwise. I never set foot in the health food section of the grocery store before, and now I'm in there all the time. It has totally changed the way we cook and eat. There's no white bread in my house anymore! We've just learned to live without it. I've replaced vegetable oil with olive oil, and we eat the Kashi crackers consistently.

"I also picked up some new tricks, like using fat-free chicken broth as a base. When I make a salad, instead of using plain old iceberg lettuce, I use spring mix and dark green, leafy vegetables.

"Others have noticed that I'm getting thinner and told me my pants are fitting better. My daughter has also lost a few pounds and gotten some comments on her weight loss.

"The best thing about the whole experience is that it works. And it's not that big of a deal—I don't feel like I'm on a diet, because it's so easy!"

DAY 26 **PECAN DAY**

BREAKFAST

Apple-Pecan Oatmeal (page 141)

OR

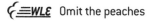 ¾ cup fat-free plain yogurt with ¼ cup low-fat pecan granola

MIDMORNING SNACK

4 pecan halves and 2 dried figs

LUNCH

Pecan, Lentil, and Tomato Mixed Greens Salad (page 169)

MIDAFTERNOON SNACK

6 pecan halves and 1 fresh peach or ½ cup canned unsweetened peaches

OR

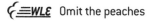 Omit the peaches

DINNER FOR 4

Pecan-Crusted Chicken (page 192)

4 cups cooked bulgur wheat (page 228)

Roasted Asparagus with Pecans and Sun-Dried Tomatoes (page 226)

Tossed Garden Salad (page 211)

DESSERT FOR 4 (OPTIONAL)

Baked Bananas with Rum-Pecan Topping (page 230)

OR

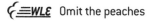 No dessert

---

Daily Nutrition Facts

REGULAR

1,479 calories: 36% from fat (4% from sat fat), 16% from protein, 47% from carbohydrate; 42 g fiber, 64 mg cholesterol, 1,035 mg sodium

WEIGHT-LOSS EXPRESS

1,226 calories: 38% from fat (5% from sat fat), 19% from protein, 43% from carbohydrate; 34 g fiber, 67 mg cholesterol, 1,123 mg sodium

DAY 27 **DILL DAY**

BREAKFAST

Asparagus and Dill Cheese Omelet (page 148)

1 slice whole grain toast, plain or with 1 tsp Smart Balance spread

OR

≡WLE 1 slice whole wheat bread with ½ chopped tomato, ½ tsp dried dill, and 1 Tbsp grated part-skim mozzarella, melted

MIDMORNING SNACK

Up to 18 baby carrots with Dill Yogurt Dip (page 154)

LUNCH

Dill Chicken Salad Sandwich (page 177) on whole grain bread

OR

≡WLE Replace the bread with 2 pieces Old London Whole Wheat Melba Toast

MIDAFTERNOON SNACK

6 Snyder's of Hanover Oat Bran Sticks with 2 Tbsp hummus mixed with a pinch of dried dill

DINNER FOR 4

Poached Salmon with Cucumber-Dill Sauce (page 207)

Dill Potatoes (page 224)

Tossed Garden Salad (page 211)

DESSERT FOR 4 (OPTIONAL)

Fruit salad (1 sliced banana; 2 medium apples, cored and cut into small chunks; and 24 grapes); ¾ cup per person

Daily Nutrition Facts

REGULAR

1,492 calories: 25% from fat (6% from sat fat), 26% from protein, 46% from carbohydrate; 37 g fiber, 528 mg cholesterol, 2,570 mg sodium

WEIGHT-LOSS EXPRESS

1,236 calories: 21% from fat (4% from sat fat), 26% from protein, 49% from carbohydrate; 28 g fiber, 167 mg cholesterol, 2,067 mg sodium

DAY 28 **CRANBERRY DAY**

BREAKFAST

2 Cranberry-Banana Soft Wheat Muffins (page 143)

1 cup fat-free milk

OR

⟨≡*WLE* Cranberry-Banana Smoothie (page 150)

MIDMORNING SNACK

$\frac{1}{2}$ cup fat-free plain yogurt with 2 tsp dried cranberries and 1 Tbsp low-fat granola

LUNCH

Cranberry-Lentil Mixed Greens Salad with Feta and Pecans (page 168)

MIDAFTERNOON SNACK

Cranberry-Banana Smoothie (page 150)

DINNER FOR 4

Cranberry and Sweet Onion Turkey Cutlets (page 197)

Baked sweet potatoes (wrap 2 whole sweet potatoes in aluminum foil and bake at 375°F until tender; unwrap and cut each in half for 1 serving)

Tossed Garden Salad (page 211; add 2 tsp dried cranberries)

DESSERT FOR 4 (OPTIONAL)

Cranberry-Vanilla Soft Ice Cream (page 243)

OR

⟨≡*WLE* No dessert

Daily Nutrition Facts

REGULAR

1,453 calories: 20% from fat (3% from sat fat), 23% from protein, 57% from carbohydrate; 24 g fiber, 150 mg cholesterol, 1,272 mg sodium

REGULAR

1,272 calories: 17% from fat (3% from sat fat), 23% from protein, 60% from carbohydrate; 24 g fiber, 117 mg cholesterol, 1,062 mg sodium

PHASE 2: **WEEKS 5 AND 6**

DAY 29

BREAKFAST

1 cup whole grain cereal with ½ cup fat-free milk

¾ cup 100% orange juice

OR

 Orange-Banana Smoothie (page 151)

MIDMORNING SNACK

4 large strawberries with Sweet Cinnamon Yogurt Dip (page 158)

LUNCH

Red Onion, White Bean, Lentil, and Tomato Salad (page 171)

4 Stacy's Simply Naked Baked Pita Chips

OR

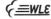 Omit the beans and chips and add 1 tomato

MIDAFTERNOON SNACK

Up to 18 baby carrots with ½ cup fat-free cottage cheese

DINNER FOR 4

 Pistachio-Crusted Chicken (page 187)

4 cups cooked bulgur wheat (page 228)

Sautéed Spaghetti Squash (page 225)

Tossed Garden Salad (page 211; add 3 Tbsp shelled pistachios)

DESSERT FOR 4 (OPTIONAL)

Peanut Katz Flax Crisps (page 238); 1 square per person

Daily Nutrition Facts

REGULAR

1,446 calories: 26% from fat (4% from sat fat), 21% from protein, 53% from carbohydrate; 37 g fiber, 72 mg cholesterol, 1,745 mg sodium

WEIGHT-LOSS EXPRESS

1,239 calories: 29% from fat (4% from sat fat), 21% from protein, 51% from carbohydrate; 27 g fiber, 70 mg cholesterol, 1,266 mg sodium

DAY 30

BREAKFAST

Mushroom, Thyme, and Cheese Omelet (page 149)

1 slice whole grain toast, plain or with 1 tsp Smart Balance spread

MIDMORNING SNACK

$^{1}/_{2}$ cup fat-free plain yogurt with 1 sliced small apple

OR

≡WLE Omit the yogurt

LUNCH

Dill Chicken Salad Sandwich (page 177) on whole grain bread

OR

≡WLE Replace the bread with 2 pieces Old London Whole Wheat Melba Toast

MIDAFTERNOON SNACK

1 cucumber cut into strips

$^{1}/_{2}$ cup fat-free cottage cheese

OR

≡WLE Omit the cottage cheese

DINNER FOR 4

Portobello Mushrooms with Walnut Stuffing (page 220)

12 oz sautéed baby spinach with 1 Tbsp chopped walnuts

Lentil and Bean Salad with Cilantro (page 213) over mixed greens

DESSERT FOR 4 (OPTIONAL)

Baked Cinnamon Apples (page 231)

Daily Nutrition Facts

REGULAR

1,478 calories: 24% from fat (6% from sat fat), 24% from protein, 52% from carbohydrate; 48 g fiber, 430 mg cholesterol, 2,429 mg sodium

WEIGHT-LOSS EXPRESS

1,265 calories: 28% from fat (7% from sat fat), 22% from protein, 50% from carbohydrate; 38 g fiber, 423 mg cholesterol, 1,845 mg sodium

DAY 31

BREAKFAST

2 slices Almond French Toast with Sliced Strawberries (page 140)

OR

⋲≡*WLE* 1 slice whole grain toast with 1 Tbsp almond butter

MIDMORNING SNACK

½ cup fat-free plain yogurt with 1 Tbsp chopped walnuts and 1 Tbsp raisins

OR

⋲≡*WLE* Omit the yogurt and replace the raisins with 1 dried apricot

LUNCH

Turkey sandwich with basil, lettuce, and tomato (2 slices whole grain bread, 2 slices unprocessed roast turkey, 2 tsp basil pesto spread, lettuce, and ½ sliced tomato)

MIDAFTERNOON SNACK

18 baked corn tortilla chips with ⅓ cup salsa

OR

⋲≡*WLE* 3 cups air-popped popcorn

DINNER FOR 4

Baked Tilapia with Tomatoes, Olives, and Capers (page 202)

4 cups cooked bulgur wheat (page 228)

10 oz sautéed fresh or frozen cauliflower florets

Tossed Garden Salad (page 211)

DESSERT FOR 4 (OPTIONAL)

Amaretto strawberry salad (3 cups sliced strawberries, 4 tsp amaretto liqueur, and 4 tsp chopped almonds); ¾ cup per person

---

Daily Nutrition Facts

REGULAR

1,474 calories: 26% from fat (5% from sat fat), 22% from protein, 52% from carbohydrate; 48 g fiber, 293 mg cholesterol, 2,533 mg sodium

WEIGHT-LOSS EXPRESS

1,243 calories: 28% from fat (4% from sat fat), 22% from protein, 49% from carbohydrate; 43 g fiber, 111 mg cholesterol, 2,041 mg sodium

DAY 32

BREAKFAST

Spinach and Feta Omelet (page 149)

1 slice whole grain toast, plain or with 1 tsp Smart Balance spread

OR

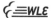 1 slice whole grain bread with 1 soft-cooked egg, 1 slice tomato, ½ tsp olive oil, and ½ Tbsp grated part-skim mozzarella, melted

MIDMORNING SNACK

1 cup fresh or canned unsweetened pineapple chunks

OR

 10 oz pineapple fizz (6 oz seltzer water and 4 oz 100% pineapple juice)

LUNCH

Stuffed Tomato with Thyme Tuna Salad (page 174)

5 Kashi TLC Original 7-Grain Crackers

OR

 Omit the crackers

MIDAFTERNOON SNACK

½ cup fat-free plain yogurt with 12 whole almonds

DINNER FOR 4

 Pumpkin Soup (page 223)

2 slices whole grain bread per person

Tossed Garden Salad (page 211; add 2 cups rinsed and drained chickpeas)

OR

 Omit 1 slice of bread

DESSERT FOR 4 (OPTIONAL)

Raisin-Granola Parfait (page 240)

Daily Nutrition Facts

REGULAR

1,492 calories: 21% from fat (5% from sat fat), 22% from protein, 57% from carbohydrate; 45 g fiber, 397 mg cholesterol, 2,567 mg sodium

WEIGHT-LOSS EXPRESS

1,225 calories: 21% from fat (4% from sat fat), 23% from protein, 56% from carbohydrate; 37 g fiber, 213 mg cholesterol, 1,941 mg sodium

DAY 33

BREAKFAST

1 cup whole grain cereal with ½ cup fat-free milk

1 fresh peach or ½ cup canned unsweetened peaches

OR

WLE Peach-Banana Smoothie (page 151)

MIDMORNING SNACK

½ cup fat-free plain yogurt with 1 sliced orange

OR

WLE Omit the yogurt

LUNCH

Lemon Tabbouleh Salad (page 167)

MIDAFTERNOON SNACK

1 bell pepper cut into strips with 2 Tbsp hummus

DINNER FOR 4 (OPTIONAL)

Carrot Cider–Glazed Chicken (page 180)

4 cups cooked bulgur wheat (page 228)

1 lb sautéed fresh or frozen broccoli rabe

Tossed Garden Salad (page 211; make with ½ cup grated carrots)

DESSERT FOR 6 (OPTIONAL)

Peach Flat Cake (page 235)

OR

WLE 1 seasonal fresh fruit per person

Daily Nutrition Facts

REGULAR

1,443 calories: 22% from fat (4% from sat fat), 19% from protein, 58% from carbohydrate; 46 g fiber, 154 mg cholesterol, 1,624 mg sodium

WEIGHT-LOSS EXPRESS

1,283 calories: 19% from fat (4% from sat fat), 19% from protein, 62% from carbohydrate; 41 g fiber, 93 mg cholesterol, 1,282 mg sodium

DAY 34

BREAKFAST

1 cup whole grain cereal with ¹/₂ cup fat-free milk

³/₄ cup 100% orange juice

OR

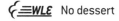 Orange-Banana Smoothie (page 151)

MIDMORNING SNACK

1 apple

LUNCH

Currant-Lentil Spinach Salad with Feta and Walnuts (page 168)

MIDAFTERNOON SNACK

Up to 18 baby carrots

DINNER FOR 4

Poppy Seed–Crusted Salmon (page 208)

4 cups cooked quinoa (page 229)

1 lb sautéed zucchini topped with 1 tsp poppy seeds

Tossed Garden Salad (page 211)

DESSERT FOR 4 (OPTIONAL)

Mixed-berry salad (1 cup each fresh blueberries, raspberries, and black-berries); ³/₄ cup per person

OR

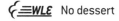 No dessert

---

Daily Nutrition Facts

REGULAR

1,498 calories: 29% from fat (4% from sat fat), 20% from protein, 51% from carbohy-drate; 38 g fiber, 115 mg cholesterol, 1,122 mg sodium

WEIGHT-LOSS EXPRESS

1,334 calories: 32% from fat (5% from sat fat), 20% from protein, 48% from carbohy-drate; 27 g fiber, 113 mg cholesterol, 886 mg sodium

DAY 35

BREAKFAST

1 cup whole grain cereal with ½ cup fat-free milk

¾ cup 100% pineapple juice

OR

 Pineapple Smoothie (page 151)

MIDMORNING SNACK

½ cup fat-free plain yogurt

½ cup unsweetened applesauce

OR

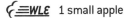 1 small apple

LUNCH

Peanut-Cucumber Salad (page 170)

MIDAFTERNOON SNACK

6 Snyder's of Hanover Oat Bran Sticks with 2 Tbsp hummus

DINNER FOR 4

Apple-Prune Chicken (page 196)

4 cups cooked bulgur wheat (page 228)

12 oz sautéed spinach

Tossed Garden Salad (page 211)

DESSERT FOR 4 (OPTIONAL)

Fruit salad (2 cups cubed cantaloupe, 2 cups cubed honeydew, and 1½ cups fresh or frozen raspberries); 1⅓ cups per person

---

Daily Nutrition Facts

REGULAR

1,432 calories: 17% from fat (3% from sat fat), 19% from protein, 64% from carbohydrate; 46 g fiber, 80 mg cholesterol, 1,688 mg sodium

WEIGHT-LOSS EXPRESS

1,272 calories: 19% from fat (3% from sat fat), 18% from protein, 64% from carbohydrate; 42 g fiber, 76 mg cholesterol, 1,377 mg sodium

DAY 36

BREAKFAST

Apple Multigrain Pancakes with Honey Yogurt Sauce (page 146)

OR

 Apple-Banana Smoothie (page 150)

MIDMORNING SNACK

½ cup fat-free fruit yogurt with 1 Tbsp chopped pecans

LUNCH

Tomato and Black Bean Mediterranean Salad (page 173) in ½ whole wheat pita

OR

 Omit the pita

MIDAFTERNOON SNACK

10 Kashi TLC Original 7-Grain Crackers with Spinach Yogurt Dip (page 158)

DINNER FOR 4

CN? Orange Cod (page 204)

1 lb sautéed fresh or frozen French-cut string beans with grated orange peel

4 cups cooked bulgur wheat (page 228)

Tossed Garden Salad (page 211; add juice of ½ orange)

DESSERT FOR 4 (OPTIONAL)

Peanut Katz Flax Crisps (page 238); 1 square per person

Daily Nutrition Facts

REGULAR

1,445 calories: 27% from fat (4% from sat fat), 19% from protein, 55% from carbohydrate; 38 g fiber, 85 mg cholesterol, 1,572 mg sodium

WEIGHT-LOSS EXPRESS

1,294 calories: 26% from fat (4% from sat fat), 17% from protein, 57% from carbohydrate; 34 g fiber, 39 mg cholesterol, 1,099 mg sodium

DAY 37

BREAKFAST

Apple-Pecan Oatmeal (page 141)

OR

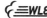 ³/₄ cup fat-free plain yogurt with ¼ cup low-fat pecan granola

MIDMORNING SNACK

1 orange

LUNCH

Roasted pepper, avocado, and hummus sandwich (2 slices whole grain bread, 2 oz roasted bell peppers, 3 Tbsp hummus, ¼ ripe black avocado, and alfalfa sprouts to taste)

OR

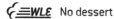 Omit the avocado

MIDAFTERNOON SNACK

12 cherry tomatoes

DINNER FOR 4

Turkey, Bean, and Thyme Pot au Feu (page 200)

4 cups cooked bulgur wheat (page 228)

Tossed Garden Salad (page 211)

DESSERT FOR 4 (OPTIONAL)

Fruit salad (1 sliced banana; 2 medium apples, cored and cut into small chunks; and 24 grapes); ³/₄ cup per person

OR

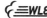 No dessert

---

Daily Nutrition Facts

REGULAR

1,501 calories: 17% from fat (2% from sat fat), 22% from protein, 59% from carbohydrate; 53 g fiber, 106 mg cholesterol, 1,462 mg sodium

WEIGHT-LOSS EXPRESS

1,274 calories: 13% from fat (2% from sat fat), 25% from protein, 59% from carbohydrate; 45 g fiber, 109 mg cholesterol, 1,547 mg sodium

DAY 38

BREAKFAST

1 slice whole grain cinnamon toast with 2 tsp almond or natural peanut butter and 3 slices banana (about $1/4$ banana)

$3/4$ cup fat-free milk

MIDMORNING SNACK

$1/2$ cup fat-free plain yogurt with 1 Tbsp chopped walnuts and 1 Tbsp raisins

OR

WLE Omit the yogurt and replace the raisins with 1 dried apricot

LUNCH

Stuffed Tomato with Thyme Tuna Salad (page 174)

5 Kashi TLC Original 7-Grain Crackers

OR

WLE Omit the crackers

MIDAFTERNOON SNACK

12 baby carrots with $1/3$ cup salsa

DINNER FOR 4

Shrimp Pasta Primavera with Basil Pesto (page 209)

Tossed Garden Salad (page 211; add fresh basil to taste)

DESSERT FOR 4 (OPTIONAL)

1 seasonal fresh fruit per person

OR

WLE No dessert

Daily Nutrition Facts

REGULAR

1,444 calories: 31% from fat (4% from sat fat), 21% from protein, 48% from carbohydrate; 30 g fiber, 124 mg cholesterol, 1,791 mg sodium

WEIGHT-LOSS EXPRESS

1,273 calories: 35% from fat (5% from sat fat), 22% from protein, 44% from carbohydrate; 27 g fiber, 121 mg cholesterol, 1,655 mg sodium

DAY 39

BREAKFAST

1 cup whole grain cereal with $\frac{1}{2}$ cup fat-free milk

1 fresh peach or $\frac{1}{2}$ cup canned unsweetened peaches

MIDMORNING SNACK

$\frac{3}{4}$ cup fat-free fruit yogurt (flavor of choice)

OR

WLE $\frac{1}{2}$ cup fat-free plain yogurt with 1 sliced orange

LUNCH

Currant-Lentil Spinach Salad with Feta and Walnuts (page 168)

MIDAFTERNOON SNACK

Up to 18 baby carrots with $\frac{1}{2}$ cup fat-free cottage cheese

OR

WLE Omit the cottage cheese

DINNER FOR 4

Honey Curry–Glazed Chicken (page 191)

1 lb sautéed fresh or frozen broccoli florets with a pinch of mild curry powder

2 cups cooked brown rice (page 228)

Tossed Garden Salad (page 211)

DESSERT FOR 4 (OPTIONAL)

Baked Cinnamon-Walnut Apples (page 231)

OR

WLE No dessert

Daily Nutrition Facts

REGULAR

1,515 calories: 22% from fat (4% from sat fat), 23% from protein, 55% from carbohydrate; 33 g fiber, 146 mg cholesterol, 1,835 mg sodium

WEIGHT-LOSS EXPRESS

1,281 calories: 22% from fat (4% from sat fat), 23% from protein, 56% from carbohydrate; 34 g fiber, 132 mg cholesterol, 1,367 mg sodium

DAY 40

BREAKFAST

$^3/_4$ cup fat-free plain yogurt with $^1/_4$ cup low-fat pecan granola and 1 cup (about 25) grapes

OR

WLE Omit the grapes

MIDMORNING SNACK

$^1/_2$ cup canned unsweetened peaches

LUNCH

Dill Chicken Salad Sandwich (page 177) on whole grain bread

OR

WLE Replace the bread with 2 pieces Old London Whole Wheat Melba Toast

MIDAFTERNOON SNACK

$^1/_2$ cup fat-free plain yogurt with 6 whole almonds

DINNER FOR 4

Pasta Fagioli with Spinach Marinara Sauce (page 215)

Tossed Garden Salad (page 211; make with spinach)

DESSERT FOR 4 (OPTIONAL)

Amaretto strawberry salad (3 cups sliced strawberries, 4 tsp amaretto liqueur, and 4 tsp chopped almonds); $^3/_4$ cup per person

---

Daily Nutrition Facts

REGULAR

1,469 calories: 18% from fat (3% from sat fat), 18% from protein, 64% from carbohydrate; 48 g fiber, 59 mg cholesterol, 1,997 mg sodium

WEIGHT-LOSS EXPRESS

1,298 calories: 20% from fat (3% from sat fat), 19% from protein, 60% from carbohydrate; 37 g fiber, 59 mg cholesterol, 1,918 mg sodium

DAY 41

BREAKFAST

2 Banana–Chocolate Chip Soft Wheat Muffins (page 143)

MIDMORNING SNACK

$1/2$ cup fat-free plain yogurt with 3 dried apricots

OR

≡WLE Omit the yogurt

LUNCH

Black Bean, Corn, and Tomato Salad (page 165) in $1/2$ whole wheat pita

OR

≡WLE Omit the pita

MIDAFTERNOON SNACK

18 baked corn tortilla chips with $1/3$ cup salsa

OR

≡WLE 3 cups air-popped popcorn

DINNER FOR 4

Pan-Seared Tilapia with Lemon Chives and Capers (page 203)

1 lb sautéed fresh or frozen asparagus with grated lemon peel

Baked fries (bake 1 bag Alexia frozen julienne fries according to package directions)

Tossed Garden Salad (page 211; add juice of 1 lemon)

DESSERT FOR 4 (OPTIONAL)

4 cups fresh blueberries with lemon peel; 1 cup per person

Daily Nutrition Facts

REGULAR

1,449 calories: 28% from fat (4% from sat fat), 18% from protein, 54% from carbohydrate; 35 g fiber, 115 mg cholesterol, 1,822 mg sodium

WEIGHT-LOSS EXPRESS

1,294 calories: 30% from fat (5% from sat fat), 18% from protein, 52% from carbohydrate; 35 g fiber, 113 mg cholesterol, 1,424 mg sodium

DAY 42

BREAKFAST

Green Scallion and Cheese Omelet (page 149)

1 slice whole grain toast, plain or with 1 tsp Smart Balance spread

MIDMORNING SNACK

Pineapple Smoothie (page 151)

LUNCH

Tuna salad sandwich (2 slices whole grain bread with tuna salad on page 174)

OR

 Stuffed Tomato with Thyme Tuna Salad (page 174)

5 Kashi TLC Original 7-Grain Crackers

MIDAFTERNOON SNACK

Up to 18 baby carrots with ½ cup fat-free cottage cheese

DINNER FOR 4

Mexican Stuffed Bell Peppers (page 193)

1 lb sautéed frozen whole-kernel sweet corn

Tossed Garden Salad (page 211)

DESSERT FOR 4 (OPTIONAL)

Baked Bananas with Rum-Pecan Topping (page 230)

OR

1 seasonal fresh fruit per person

Daily Nutrition Facts

REGULAR

1,506 calories: 23% from fat (5% from sat fat), 23% from protein, 54% from carbohydrate; 42 g fiber, 447 mg cholesterol, 2,584 mg sodium

WEIGHT-LOSS EXPRESS

1,343 calories: 22% from fat (6% from sat fat), 25% from protein, 53% from carbohydrate; 33 g fiber, 447 mg cholesterol, 2,489 mg sodium

SPECIAL INDULGENCE DAY **CHOCOLATE DAY**

BREAKFAST

1 Banana–Chocolate Chip Soft Wheat Muffin (page 143)

6 oz hot cocoa (6 oz hot fat-free milk with 2 Tbsp Ghirardelli sweet ground chocolate and cocoa)

MIDMORNING SNACK

Chocolate chip trail mix (1 Tbsp raisins, 1 Tbsp semisweet chocolate chips, and 3 whole almonds)

LUNCH

Chocolate and Banana Grilled Panini (page 178)

1 cup fat-free milk

MIDAFTERNOON SNACK

Strawberries Dipped in Dark Chocolate (page 241)

DINNER FOR 4

Chicken with Chocolate Port Wine Sauce (page 182)

1 lb sautéed fresh baby spinach

DESSERT FOR 4 (OPTIONAL)

Chocolate Brownies (page 232); 1 brownie per person

Daily Nutrition Facts

1,500 calories: 28% from fat (11% from sat fat), 20% from protein, 49% from carbohydrate; 29 g fiber, 146 mg cholesterol, 1,537 mg sodium

SPECIAL INDULGENCE DAY **COCONUT DAY**

BREAKFAST

Coconut-Pineapple Smoothie (page 150)

MIDMORNING SNACK

Coconut trail mix (2 Tbsp raisins, 1 Tbsp unsweetened shredded coconut, and 3 whole almonds)

LUNCH

Coconut Shrimp and Avocado Salad (page 164)

MIDAFTERNOON SNACK

1 cup fat-free plain yogurt with 5 sliced large strawberries and 1 Tbsp unsweetened shredded coconut

DINNER FOR 4

Coconut Thai Chicken (page 186)

3 cups cooked brown rice (page 228)

1 lb sautéed snap peas

Tossed Garden Salad (page 211)

DESSERT FOR 4 (OPTIONAL)

Piña Colada Frozen Dessert (page 238)

Daily Nutrition Facts

1,517 calories: 31% from fat (9% from sat fat), 18% from protein, 50% from carbohydrate; 26 g fiber, 138 mg cholesterol, 1,592 mg sodium

FLAVOR-FRIENDLY ALTERNATIVES

Any day of the week in any phase of the plan, feel free to replace the breakfast, snacks, or lunch on the menu with one of the flavor-friendly options on the following pages. For best results, use the brands specified on these pages. If you can't find those brands at your store, be sure your breakfast cereal, waffles, bread, and crackers have at least 2 grams of fiber per 100 calories, no trans fats (that means no partially hydrogenated oil), and no high-fructose corn syrup. Jam should have no added sugar or high-fructose corn syrup.

BREAKFAST OPTIONS

BREAKFAST #1

1¹/₂ cups whole grain cereal with ³/₄ cup fat-free milk

Choose from the following cereals.

NATURE'S PATH

Organic Heritage Flakes

Organic Multigrain Oat Bran Flakes

HEALTH VALLEY

Organic Blue Corn Flakes

Organic Healthy Fiber Multigrain Flakes

KASHI

GoLean

Heart to Heart

Nutritional analysis (on average) per serving: 269 calories; 2 g fat (0 g sat fat), 15 g protein, 56 g carbohydrate, 11 g fiber; 3 mg cholesterol, 245 mg sodium

BREAKFAST #2

2 slices whole grain bread or 2 Van's All-Natural Belgian 7-Grain Waffles, plain or with 2 tsp Smart Balance spread or 2 tsp all-fruit jam (matching the flavor theme of the day)

1 cup fat-free milk

Choose from the following breads.

ALVARADO STREET BAKERY

Sprouted Rye Seed

VERMONT BREAD COMPANY

Whole Wheat

Sprouted Whole Wheat

Soft Whole Wheat

NATURAL OVENS

Right Wheat

100% Whole Grain

Multigrain

Nutritional analysis (on average) per serving: 236 calories, 3 g fat (1 g sat fat), 15 g protein, 42 g carbohydrate, 7 g fiber, 5 mg cholesterol, 385 mg sodium

BREAKFAST #3

1 bowl of oatmeal (page 141), plain or with $1/4$ cup fat-free fruit yogurt or $1/2$ cup fresh fruit (matching the flavor theme of the day)

Nutritional analysis (on average) per serving: 291 calories, 56 g fat (1 g sat fat), 13 g protein, 53 g carbohydrate, 6 g fiber, 2 mg cholesterol, 74 mg sodium

BREAKFAST #4

2 eggs (organic, with omega-3's), soft-cooked, scrambled, or over easy (cook in a nonstick skillet coated with olive oil spray)

2 slices whole grain toast, plain or with 1 tsp Smart Balance spread

Choose from the suggested bread brands listed for Breakfast #2.

Nutritional analysis (on average) per serving: 281 calories, 12 g fat (3 g sat fat), 19 g protein, 26 g carbohydrate, 7 g fiber, 360 mg cholesterol, 388 mg sodium

MIDMORNING SNACK OPTIONS

SNACK

$1/2$ cup fat-free plain yogurt with $1/4$ cup whole grain cereal

Choose from the following cereals.

NATURE'S PATH

Organic Heritage Flakes

Organic Multigrain Oat Bran Flakes

HEALTH VALLEY

Organic Blue Corn Flakes

Organic Healthy Fiber Multigrain Flakes

KASHI

GoLean

Heart to Heart

BARBARA'S BAKERY

Bite-Size Shredded Oats

Organic Crispy Wheats

POST

Spoon-Size Shredded Wheat 'N Bran

Nutritional analysis (on average) per serving: 86 calories, 0 g fat (0 g sat fat), 6 g protein, 18 g carbohydrate, 2 g fiber, 3 mg cholesterol, 96 mg sodium

LUNCH OPTIONS

SALAD

1–2 cups of favorite mixed greens or lettuce (preferably not iceberg)

As many raw vegetables as you can pile on—tomatoes, cucumbers, onions, bell pepper strips, alfalfa sprouts, and so on. (For ease and convenience, use packaged, prewashed shredded carrots, shredded cabbage-carrot coleslaw, or shredded broccoli-cabbage coleslaw.)

A drizzle of olive oil ($1^1/_2$ tsp) and vinegar (1 Tbsp) and a pinch of salt and pepper or no more than 2 Tbsp (2 capfuls) Newman's Own Light Italian Dressing

Choose from the following toppings.

3 slices plain, unprocessed roasted deli turkey breast (no saturated fat or added sugar)

3 oz grilled chicken cutlet (in a cast-iron skillet with olive oil spray)

4 oz grilled tilapia fillet (in a nonstick skillet with olive oil spray)

3 oz drained water-packed tuna

1 hard-cooked egg and 1sliced egg white

$^1/_3$ cup rinsed and drained chickpeas or beans

Nutritional analysis (on average) per serving: 278 calories, 10 g fat (2 g sat fat), 21 g protein, 29 g carbohydrate, 9 g fiber, 59 mg cholesterol, 411 mg sodium

MIDAFTERNOON SNACK OPTIONS

SNACKS

2 Tbsp plain hummus with your choice of either 1 to 2 cups of the following raw veggies in any combination or any of the following crackers in the amount specified.

VEGETABLES

Cauliflower florets

Sliced celery

Sliced cucumber

Edamame (a small handful after shelling)

Green beans

Chopped Romaine lettuce

Snap peas

CRACKERS

2 Ak-Mak 100% Whole Wheat Sesame Crackers

10 GeniSoy Deep Sea Salt Soy Crisps

5 Kashi TLC Original 7-Grain Crackers

5 Old London Whole Wheat Melba Snacks

3 Old London Whole Wheat Melba Toasts

6 Snyder's of Hanover Oat Bran Sticks

2 Wasa Light Rye or Hearty Rye Crispbreads

Nutritional analysis (on average) per serving: 98 calories, 3 g fat (0 g sat fat), 3 g protein, 15 g carbohydrate, 3 g fiber, 0 mg cholesterol, 170 mg sodium

DINNER OPTIONS

Whole roasted chicken (skin removed) from the supermarket

OR

4 chicken cutlets (4 oz each) or 4 tilapia or cod fillets (5 oz each)

Heat 2 to 3 tsp olive oil in a cast-iron grill pan for chicken or a nonstick skillet for fish (lightly dust fish with whole grain flour). Grill or cook for 3 to 4 minutes on each side and season with a pinch of salt and pepper.

4 cups cooked bulgur wheat (page 228)

Tossed Garden Salad (page 211)

Nutritional analysis (on average) per serving, with chicken: 463 calories, 8 g fat (<2 g sat fat), 45 g protein, 53 g carbohydrate, 15 g fiber, 96 mg cholesterol, 212 mg sodium (not counting any added to chicken)

With fish: 421 calories, 7 g fat (<2 g sat fat), 40 g protein, 53 g carbohydrate, 15 g fiber, 65 mg cholesterol, 194 mg sodium (not counting any added to fish)

Satisfaction at the Flavor Point

THE FLAVOR FACTS

Name: Janet Mazur

Age: 50

Hometown: Shelton, Connecticut

Family status: Married with two children, ages 16 and 20

Occupation: Medical biller

Starting weight: 198

Pounds lost: 16 in 12 weeks

Health stats: Blood pressure dropped 10 points; cholesterol dropped 48 points; waist measurement shrank 2 inches; 4 percent decline in body fat

"This program came at the perfect time in my life. My brother was recently diagnosed with diabetes, and due to my age and weight of 198 pounds, I was also at high risk. I knew it was time to do something.

"As it turned out, the program is perfect for me because I was looking for something that would help me lose weight and improve my overall health at the same time. I had tried Weight Watchers in the past, and it didn't work at all. It became more of a social hour, and some of the partic-

ipants were fanatical. For instance, if I wore jeans to the meeting, they'd scold me because 'jeans add weight.' One woman wore the exact same outfit to every meeting to get weighed in—it was crazy. Plus, I only lost 6 pounds.

"But Dr. Katz's program is a completely different story. I feel so much better on it. The first few weeks were a little challenging, but then everything just fell into place; now I look at food in a totally different way.

"The best thing is that I have so much more energy! I used to come home from work and immediately sit down and read the paper. Now I'm bouncing around and doing things. Plus, I've been using my exercise bike for a half hour each day.

"As far as preparation is concerned, if you're organized, the recipes are really quick and easy. You buy the fish, throw half in the freezer, and you're set for the rest of the week.

"I enjoy almost all the dishes, as does my family. And it's simple to work around the program—if my family doesn't want the bulgur wheat or sweet potatoes, I make them brown rice or regular mashed potatoes as a side dish and stick to the program myself.

"My personal favorite recipe is the Mexican Stuffed Bell Peppers, and it's great that I can use the stuffing as a dip for vegetables as well. I also love the stewed turkey—it's so tender and wonderful on top of the bulgur wheat. And the tilapia and cod and turkey cutlets are also high on my list of favorites.

"It was also an easy program to customize to my life. I went out for dinner a few times and just ordered fish with steamed vegetables or a salad with chicken. Luckily, most restaurants have a number of healthful choices on their menus now, which helps.

"The snack foods on the program not only help keep me from feeling hungry, they're enjoyable as well. When I want something to munch on at 2 in the afternoon, I have plenty of options (and they're the *right* options!). So now, instead of reaching for empty calories (like a candy bar) during the day, I drink a glass of water or go for one of the snacks on the program. I love the chips and salsa, unsweetened applesauce, yogurt, and pretzels. And the seltzer with pineapple juice is delicious!

"I used to be a big sweet eater, but now I have to scrape frosting off a piece of cake because it tastes too sweet to me. If a strong urge for something sweet strikes, I eat a piece of dark chocolate, half a cookie, or 2 tablespoons of ice cream, and that's enough to quell it.

"The best part is, I'm seeing results. A lot of people have noticed my weight loss, telling me I look skinnier and that I have more color in my face. I had to buy two new pairs of pants, and I think I'm going to have to buy yet another size smaller soon. I pulled an old pair of pants out of my closet that I couldn't wear for years and was happily able to button them!

"Even though my 12 weeks are over, I'm definitely going to stick with Dr. Katz's program." ■

THE FLAVOR POINT
DIET RECIPES

More than 100 options that are so delicious, you won't believe they're this good for you.

Many times over the years, I have heard people lament, "If it tastes good, it's bad for you!" I've already discussed the hidden significance of how we register taste. Now, let's attack this regret head-on by noting, quite bluntly: It doesn't have to be that way!

Diets have long given weight control a deservedly bad reputation, since most of them are based on what you have to give up. Until the low-carb diets came along, diet food was often dismissively equated with rabbit (or some alternative rodent) food. True, the low-carb diets fixed this (I've never seen a rabbit eat bacon!). They did so, however, with diets that are, in my view, at odds with good health and unrealistically restrictive over the long term.

Well, folks, welcome to a new place. When I tell you that the Flavor Point Diet is based on the power of taste, I truly mean *tasty* taste! This food is, in a word, delicious.

The Flavor Point Diet recipes will show you that the joy of eating and the joy of weight loss can indeed come together at the same dinner table. I know, because it's *my* dinner table, too!

When Catherine and I married, the process of marrying my devotion to nutrition and her skill in the kitchen also began. In these recipes, you'll find the culinary offspring of this union. Like any relationship, this one took work. It took years of figuring out how to combine the very best of taste with the very best of nutrition. We did the trial and put up with some inevitable error, so now you don't have to. I really like good food and can personally vouch for every recipe in the Flavor Point Diet. I expect these flavorful yet simple recipes to become a hit with everyone in your family, just as they have in ours.

I love Catherine's Banana Soft Wheat Muffins, and so do our kids, who often bake them by themselves.

I would happily eat Black Bean, Corn, and Tomato Salad every day, except for the days when I might rather have Curry, Lentil, and Spinach Salad with Gorgonzola and Walnuts. All I can say about Almond-Crusted Tilapia is "Yum!" and in our household of seven, it's pretty much a rumble to see who can get to the Honey Curry–Glazed Chicken first. I could go on, but I trust you get the idea. This food is good!

The recipes are also convenient. For us to use them in our crazy schedules, they really have to be. Many take 15 minutes or less to prepare. Most use convenient ingredients, such as prechopped vegetables, to get you and your family to the dinner table with minimal time and effort. They all use the best, most healthful ingredients the food supply has to offer. From the types of fish to the types of vegetables used in each recipe, you will be consuming the most nutritious foods you can get. Not only will their simple, flavorful preparation help lower your Flavor Point, it will also help improve your overall health and well-being.

The Flavor Point recipes are designed to transform your whole diet, forever. Just because we've focused on the big picture doesn't mean we didn't address every detail. Each recommendation in these recipes has a rationale. We recommend wild salmon over farm-raised salmon, for example, assuming you can find and afford it. (We always say, "Don't make perfect the enemy of good!"). Wild salmon is more flavorful, relatively free of contaminating chemicals, and richer in healthful omega-3 fatty acids. We recommend natural over processed peanut butter to help you cut out unnecessary sugar, salt, and harmful trans fat. We encourage organic foods if you can afford them, both for your benefit and for that of the planet. We encourage selecting eggs that are enriched with omega-3's. In every instance, our recommendations are directed toward optimizing your shopping cart and pantry on the way to optimizing your health and weight.

Which recipes will *you* like best? I don't know. That's a matter of . . . taste! I'm quite confident that you will find many future favorites here. As you master the Flavor Point principles, I'll bet you will cook up some real winners of your own. Eating well for enjoyment, health, and lasting weight control is suited to everyone's tastes. You'll find the recipe for *that* in the recipes that follow—so *bon appétit!*

BREAKFASTS

Almond French Toast with Sliced Strawberries

Whenever you find the time to make French toast,
you'll love this recipe.

SERVES 1

1 egg
1 tablespoon fat-free milk
1 drop almond extract
2 slices whole grain bread*
2 teaspoons Smart Balance spread
$^1/_2$ teaspoon confectioners' sugar
1 teaspoon finely ground almonds
3 large strawberries, sliced

1. In a shallow bowl, whisk the egg with the milk and almond extract.

2. Dip the bread in the egg mixture, coating both sides lightly. Set aside.

3. Heat the spread in a nonstick skillet large enough to hold both pieces of bread. Add the bread and cook on medium heat for 1 to 2 minutes, then turn and cook for 1 minute.

4. To serve, dust with the confectioner's sugar and ground almonds and top with the strawberries.

Per serving: 281 calories, 13 g fat (3 g sat fat), 11 g protein, 34 g carbohydrate, 11 g fiber, 180 mg cholesterol, 294 mg sodium

*See the appendix for recommended brands.

VARIATION

Sesame French Toast with Sliced Strawberries: Sprinkle with 1

teaspoon sesame seeds instead of almonds in step 4.

Per serving: 287 calories, 13g fat (3 g sat fat), 11 g protein, 35 g carbohydrate,
12 g fiber, 180 mg cholesterol, 294 mg sodium

Apple-Raisin Oatmeal

A complete and heartwarming breakfast in a bowl!

SERVES 1

$^2/_3$ cup water

$^1/_4$ cup fat-free milk

  1 tablespoon nonfat dry milk

$^1/_2$ cup quick-cooking oats

$^1/_3$ cup unsweetened applesauce

  1 tablespoon raisins

1–2 teaspoons brown sugar (optional)

1. In a small saucepan, bring the water and milk to a boil.

2. Add the dry milk and oatmeal and cook for 1 to 2 minutes. Remove from
   the heat, cover, and let stand for 2 minutes.

3. Add the applesauce and raisins. Spoon into a bowl and sprinkle with the
   brown sugar (if using).

Per serving: 261 calories, 3 g fat (<1 g sat fat), 11 g protein, 49 g carbohydrate, 5 g fiber,
1 mg cholesterol, 68 mg sodium

VARIATION

Apple-Pecan Oatmeal: Add 2 teaspoons chopped pecans in step 3.

Per serving: 280 calories, 6 g fat (<1 g sat fat), 11 g protein, 46 g carbohydrate,
5 g fiber, 1 mg cholesterol, 67 mg sodium

Banana Soft Wheat Muffins

These muffins are filled with fiber and fruit and are very low in fat and sugar. Because the recipe replaces some of the sugar normally found in muffin recipes with milk, they offer more calcium than usual. They also freeze well, so make a batch and keep the extras for another day. This basic recipe can be modified many different ways. Use the variations to adapt the recipe to the flavor theme of the day.

MAKES 12 MUFFINS

2 medium ripe bananas

1 egg

3 tablespoons packed dark brown sugar

3 tablespoons nonfat dry milk

3 tablespoons canola oil

1 1/2 cups soft wheat pastry flour*

1 teaspoon baking powder

1/3 cup fat-free milk

1. Preheat the oven to 350°F.

2. Place the bananas, egg, brown sugar, dry milk, and oil in the bowl of an electric mixer and beat until well blended.

3. Add the flour and baking powder and beat on low, adding the milk slowly until well blended.

4. Place 12 foil baking cups on a baking sheet or line a 12-cup muffin pan with paper liners. Spoon in the batter, filling each cup 2/3 full.

5. Bake for 15 to 20 minutes, or until golden.

Per muffin: 115 calories, 4 g fat (0 g sat fat), 3 g protein, 18 g carbohydrate, 2 g fiber, 15 mg cholesterol, 50 mg sodium

*Arrowhead Mills Organic Pastry Flour or any other brand of soft wheat (not whole wheat) flour with fiber is fine. You can also use Hodgson Mill Oat Bran Flour.

VARIATIONS

Banana–Chocolate Chip Soft Wheat Muffins: Add $\frac{1}{3}$ cup Ghirardelli Double Chocolate Chips in step 4.

Per muffin: 141 calories, 6 g fat (1 g sat fat), 3 g protein, 21 g carbohydrate, 2 g fiber, 15 mg cholesterol, 50 mg sodium

Cranberry-Banana Soft Wheat Muffins: Add $\frac{1}{2}$ cup fresh or frozen cranberries in step 4.

Per muffin: 118 calories, 4 g fat (0 g sat fat), 3 g protein, 18 g carbohydrate, 2 g fiber, 15 mg cholesterol, 57 mg sodium

Pumpkin-Banana Soft Wheat Muffins

The sweet flavors of banana and pumpkin were made for each other!

MAKES 12 MUFFINS

   1 small ripe banana
 ½ cup canned pumpkin (no added salt or sugar)
   2 eggs
 ¼ cup packed dark brown sugar
 ¼ cup nonfat dry milk
   3 tablespoons canola oil
 1½ cups soft wheat pastry flour*
   1 teaspoon baking powder
 ½ cup fat-free milk
 ⅓ cup chopped pecans

1. Preheat the oven to 350°F.

2. Place the banana, pumpkin, eggs, brown sugar, dry milk, and oil in the bowl of an electric mixer and beat until well blended.

3. Add the flour and baking powder and beat on low, adding the milk slowly until well blended.

4. Place 12 foil baking cups on a baking sheet or line a 12-cup muffin pan with paper liners. Spoon in the batter, filling each cup ⅔ full.

5. Bake for 15 to 20 minutes, or until golden.

Per muffin: 141 calories, 7 g fat (<1 g sat fat), 4 g protein, 17 g carbohydrate, 2 g fiber, 30 mg cholesterol, 58 mg sodium

*Arrowhead Mills Organic Pastry Flour or any other brand of soft wheat (not whole wheat) flour with fiber is fine. You can also use Hodgson Mill Oat Bran Flour.

Lemon-Poppy Soft Wheat Muffins

Simply delicious and nutritious! These muffins freeze well, so make a batch and keep the extras for another lemon- or poppy seed–theme day.

MAKES 12 MUFFINS

- ³/₄ cup fat-free lemon yogurt*
-      Grated peel of 1 lemon
- 2 eggs
- ¹/₄ cup granulated sugar
- ¹/₄ cup nonfat dry milk
- 1 tablespoon poppy seeds
- 3 tablespoons canola oil
- 1¹/₂ cups soft wheat pastry flour†
- 1 teaspoon baking powder
- ¹/₃ cup fat-free milk

1. Preheat the oven to 350°F.

2. Place the yogurt, lemon peel, eggs, sugar, dry milk, poppy seeds, and oil in the bowl of an electric mixer and beat until creamy.

3. Add the flour and baking powder and beat on low speed, adding the milk slowly until well blended.

4. Place 12 foil baking cups on a baking sheet or line a 12-cup muffin pan with paper liners. Spoon in the batter, filling each cup ²/₃ full.

5. Bake for 15 to 20 minutes, or until golden.

Per muffin: 120 calories, 5 g fat (<1 g sat fat), 4 g protein, 16 g carbohydrate, 1 g fiber, 31 mg cholesterol, 70 mg sodium

*See the appendix for recommended brands.

†Arrowhead Mills Organic Pastry Flour or any other brand of soft wheat (not whole wheat) flour with fiber is fine. You can also use Hodgson Mill Oat Bran Flour.

Apple Multigrain Pancakes with Honey Yogurt Sauce

These pancakes are light and fluffy and just as delicious as they are nutritious, as long as you use the recommended brand of pancake mix.

SERVES 4*

- 1 apple, peeled and cored
- 1 cup Arrowhead Mills Multigrain Pancake and Waffle Mix
- $\frac{1}{4}$ cup fat-free milk
- $\frac{1}{2}$ cup water
- 1 tablespoon canola oil
- 1 egg
- 1 cup fat-free plain yogurt
- 1 teaspoon natural honey
-    Pinch of cinnamon

1. Preheat a griddle to 375° to 400°F and coat with canola oil spray. With a vegetable peeler or grater, shave the apple into a medium bowl.

2. Add the pancake mix, milk, water, oil, and egg and stir until smooth. Add the grated apple.

3. Spoon the batter in batches onto the griddle and cook until bubbles form on the surface and the edges begin to dry. Turn and cook on the other side until golden.

4. In a small bowl, stir together the yogurt, honey, and cinnamon. Serve with the pancakes.

Per serving: 222 calories, 5 g fat (<1 g sat fat), 10 g protein, 36 g carbohydrate, 4 g fiber, 46 mg cholesterol, 319 mg sodium

*Serving size: 2 (4") pancakes and $\frac{1}{4}$ cup sauce

VARIATION

Walnut Multigrain Pancakes with Honey Yogurt Sauce: Add 2 tablespoons chopped walnuts instead of the apple in step 2.

Per serving: 228 calories, 8 g fat (<1 g sat fat), 10 g protein, 32 g carbohydrate,
3 g fiber, 46 mg cholesterol, 319 mg sodium

Scrambled Eggs with Thyme

*Herbs such as thyme hint at saltiness to our taste buds
but don't add sodium to our diets.*

SERVES 1

2 eggs
1 tablespoon fat-free milk
   Pinch of salt
   Pinch of dried thyme

1. Coat a nonstick skillet with olive oil spray.

2. In a cup, stir together the eggs and milk. Add the eggs to the skillet with
   the salt and thyme and scramble over medium heat.

Per serving: 146 calories, 9 g fat (3 g sat fat), 13 g protein, 1 g carbohydrate, 0 g fiber,
360 mg cholesterol, 429 mg sodium

Bell Pepper and Cheese Omelet

Because cheese tends to provide calories and saturated fat that no one needs, we use it only in moderation in the Flavor Point Meal Plan. That said, cheese is delicious, and when used thoughtfully, it's a flavorful, high-calcium addition to the diet. As for eggs, they're an ideal protein source, and more and more research suggests that in the context of a healthy diet, cholesterol content isn't a real worry. So enjoy!

SERVES 1

2 large eggs
1 tablespoon fat-free milk
   Pinch of salt
   Pinch of garlic powder
1 tablespoon grated part-skim mozzarella cheese
2 ounces Mancini roasted sweet peppers

1. Coat a nonstick skillet with olive oil spray and place over medium heat.

2. In a small bowl, whisk the eggs, milk, salt, and garlic powder.

3. Pour the eggs into the skillet. As they start to set around the edges, use a spatula to lift the edges and tilt the pan so the uncooked egg in the middle flows around the edges. Continue until the eggs no longer flow freely.

4. Spoon the cheese and peppers onto one half of the omelet, then fold in half and cook on both sides until golden.

Per serving: 184 calories, 10 g fat (4 g sat fat), 14 g protein, 7 g carbohydrate, <1 g fiber, 364 mg cholesterol, 573 mg sodium

VARIATIONS

Asparagus and Dill Cheese Omelet: Wash and slice 3 asparagus spears. Sauté for 2 to 3 minutes in the heated skillet, then re-move and set aside. Cook the omelet as directed, then add the asparagus and a pinch of dried dill (or 1 teaspoon fresh) instead of the peppers in step 4.

Per serving: 181 calories, 11 g fat (4 g sat fat), 15 g protein, 3 g carbohydrate, <1 g fiber, 365 mg cholesterol, 437 mg sodium

Green Scallion and Cheese Omelet: Add 1 chopped scallion instead of the peppers in step 4.

Per serving: 170 calories, 10 g fat (4 g sat fat), 15 g protein, 2 g carbohydrate, 1 g fiber, 364 mg cholesterol, 319 mg sodium

Mushroom, Thyme, and Cheese Omelet: Wash and slice 4 fresh medium mushrooms. Sauté for 2 to 3 minutes in the heated skillet, then remove and set aside. Cook the omelet as directed, then add the mushrooms and a pinch of dried thyme instead of the peppers in step 4.

Per serving: 183 calories, 11 g fat (4 g sat fat), 16 g protein, 4 g carbohydrate, <1 g fiber, 365 mg cholesterol, 437 mg sodium

Spinach and Feta Omelet: Add 2 teaspoons feta cheese instead of the mozzarella and $1/2$ cup loose-leaf raw baby spinach instead of the peppers in step 4.

Per serving: 167 calories, 10 g fat (4 g sat fat), 14 g protein, 2 g carbohydrate, <1 g fiber, 366 mg cholesterol, 518 mg sodium

Tomato, Basil, and Feta Omelet: Add 2 teaspoons feta cheese instead of the mozzarella and $1/2$ chopped tomato and 5 rinsed and dried fresh basil leaves instead of the peppers in step 4.

Per serving: 173 calories, 10 fat (4 g sat fat), 14 g protein, 4 g carbohydrate, 1 g fiber, 363 mg cholesterol, 480 mg sodium

Apple-Banana Smoothie

Use the variations of this recipe to adapt it to the flavor theme of the day.

SERVES 1

$^3/_4$ cup 100% apple juice

$^1/_2$ ripe banana

1 tablespoon fat-free plain or vanilla yogurt

$^1/_2$ cup crushed ice

Place the juice, banana, yogurt, and ice in a blender and process until smooth.

Per serving: 156 calories, 0.5 g fat (0 g sat fat), 2 g protein, 38 g carbohydrate, 2 g fiber, 0 mg cholesterol, 17 mg sodium

VARIATIONS

Carrot-Pineapple Smoothie: Replace the apple juice with $^1/_2$ cup each carrot juice and pineapple juice. Omit the banana.
Per serving: 130 calories, 0 g fat (0 g sat fat), 2 g protein, 32 g carbohydrate, 1 g fiber, 0 mg cholesterol, 49 mg sodium

Coconut-Pineapple Smoothie: Use 100% pineapple juice instead of the apple juice. Replace the banana with $^1/_2$ cup drained crushed pineapple. Replace the yogurt with $^1/_4$ cup light unsweetened coconut milk.
Per serving: 208 calories, 3 g fat (3 g sat fat), 2 g protein, 45 g carbohydrate, 1 g fiber, 0 mg cholesterol, 27 mg sodium

Cranberry-Banana Smoothie: Use 100% cranberry juice instead of the apple juice and add 2 tablespoons yogurt.
Per serving: 145 calories, 0 g fat (0 g sat fat), 4 g protein, 35 g carbohydrate, 3 g fiber, 1 mg cholesterol, 34 mg sodium

Grape-Banana Smoothie: Use 100% grape juice instead of the apple juice.
Per serving: 177 calories, 0 g fat (0 g sat fat), 2 g protein, 44 g carbohydrate, 2 g fiber, 0 mg cholesterol, 14 mg sodium

Orange-Banana Smoothie: Use 100% orange juice instead of the apple juice.

Per serving: 154 calories, 0 g fat (0 g sat fat), 1 g protein, 37 g carbohydrate, 1 g fiber, 0 mg cholesterol, 31 mg sodium

Peach-Banana Smoothie: Replace the apple juice with 1 cup canned unsweetened peaches with juice.

Per serving: 170 calories, 0 g fat (0 g sat fat), 3 g protein, 43 g carbohydrate, 4 g fiber, 0 mg cholesterol, 21 mg sodium

Pineapple Smoothie

Along with its wonderful flavor and an aroma that evokes swaying palm trees and pristine beaches, pineapple provides an abundance of potassium and vitamin C and moderate amounts of fiber, folate, and calcium.

SERVES 1

1   cup fresh pineapple chunks or juice-packed canned pineapple
1   tablespoon fat-free plain yogurt
$1/2$ cup crushed ice

Place the pineapple, yogurt, and ice in a blender and process until smooth.

Per serving: 156 calories, 0 g fat (0 g sat fat), 2 g protein, 40 g carbohydrate, 2 g fiber, 0 mg cholesterol, 11 mg sodium

Lemon-Orange Smoothie

A little tart and surprisingly delicious.

SERVES 1

- ³/₄ cup fat-free lemon yogurt
- ¹/₂ cup 100% orange juice
- ¹/₄ cup fresh lemon juice
- ¹/₂ cup crushed ice

Place the yogurt, orange juice, lemon juice, and ice in a blender and process until smooth.

Per serving: 170 calories, 0 g fat (0 g sat fat), 6 g protein, 37 g carbohydrate, 0 g fiber, 4 mg cholesterol, 100 mg sodium

Pumpkin-Allspice Smoothie

This creamy smoothie has a delicious blend of flavors. It tastes like pumpkin pie!

SERVES 2

- ¹/₄ cup canned pumpkin (no added salt or sugar)
- ¹/₄ cup fat-free vanilla yogurt
- ¹/₄ cup nonfat dry milk
- ³/₄ cup fat-free milk
- ¹/₂ cup crushed ice
-       Pinch of ground allspice

Place the pumpkin, yogurt, dry milk, fat-free milk, ice, and allspice in a blender and process until smooth.

Per serving: 105 calories, 0 g fat (0 g sat fat), 9 g protein, 37 g carbohydrate, 1g fiber, 2 mg cholesterol, 122 mg sodium

Almond-Banana Smoothie

This unusual smoothie will quickly become a rich and satisfying favorite. Almonds are a great source of calcium, magnesium, potassium, and fiber as well as healthful unsaturated oils. Bananas provide plenty of potassium and fiber as well as moderate amounts of vitamin A, folate, and magnesium.

SERVES 1

1 teaspoon natural almond butter
$1/3$ ripe banana
2 tablespoons fat-free vanilla yogurt
2 tablespoons nonfat dry milk
$1/3$ cup fat-free milk
Drop of almond extract
$1/2$ cup crushed ice

1. Spread the almond butter on the tip of the banana.

2. Place the banana, yogurt, dry milk, fat-free milk, almond extract, and ice in a blender and process until smooth.

Per serving: 160 calories, 3 g fat (<1 g sat fat), 9 g protein, 25 g carbohydrate, 1 g fiber, 1 mg cholesterol, 116 mg sodium

DIPS

Basil-Ricotta Dip

We eat them only in small quantities, but herbs and spices tend to be nutritional powerhouses. For example, calorie for calorie, basil is higher in fiber than most grains, richer in calcium than spinach, and higher in potassium than a banana. It just happens to taste great, too!

SERVES 1

- ¼ cup fat-free ricotta cheese
- 10 fresh basil leaves, chopped

In a small bowl, stir together the ricotta and basil until blended. Refrigerate until ready to serve.

Per serving: 51 calories, 0 g fat (0 g sat fat), 5 g protein, 5 g carbohydrate, 0 g fiber, 10 mg cholesterol, 65 mg sodium

Dill Yogurt Dip

Dill is rich in vitamin A, calcium, and potassium.

SERVES 1

- ¼ cup fat-free plain yogurt
- 1 teaspoon fresh dill or ⅛ teaspoon dried
    Pinch of garlic powder
    Pinch of salt

In a small bowl, stir together the yogurt, dill, garlic powder, and salt until blended. Refrigerate until ready to serve.

Per serving: 26 calories, 0 g fat (0 g sat fat), 3 g protein, 5 g carbohydrate, 0 g fiber, 1 mg cholesterol, 189 mg sodium

Bell Pepper Yogurt Dip

Fat-free yogurt is a great alternative to traditional mayonnaise as a base for dips. Whereas mayonnaise provides a large load of fat and calories, yogurt provides neither of these and is a great source of calcium and those famous active cultures.

SERVES 1

$^1\!/_2$ red bell pepper, cored and seeded
$^1\!/_2$ cup fat-free plain yogurt
    Pinch of garlic powder
    Pinch of salt

Finely chop the pepper in a small food processor. In a small bowl, stir together the pepper, yogurt, garlic powder, and salt until blended. Refrigerate until ready to serve.

Per serving: 67 calories, 0 g fat (0 g sat fat), 6 g protein, 14 g carbohydrate, 1 g fiber, 2 mg cholesterol, 146 mg sodium

Mushroom Dip

Fat-free cottage cheese is a great calcium source. Mushrooms provide plenty of fiber, potassium, selenium, and vitamin D. Are we taking good care of you, or what?

SERVES 1

$1/2$ cup sliced raw mushrooms
$1/4$ cup fat-free cottage cheese
    Pinch of garlic powder
    Pinch of dried dill

1. Grind the mushrooms in a small food processor.

2. In a small bowl, stir together the cottage cheese, mushrooms, garlic powder, and dill until blended. Refrigerate until ready to serve.

Per serving: 89 calories, 0 g fat (0 g sat fat), 14 g protein, 8 g carbohydrate, 1 g fiber, 5 mg cholesterol, 442 mg sodium

Scallion Yogurt Dip

Scallions are as nutritious as they are flavorful. They're a concentrated source of vitamin K, antioxidant carotenoids, vitamin A, folate, potassium, and calcium.

SERVES 1

$1/2$ scallion
$1/4$ cup fat-free plain yogurt
$1/8$ teaspoon onion powder
Pinch of salt

1. Finely chop the scallion in a small food processor.

2. In a small bowl, stir together the scallion, yogurt, onion powder, and salt until blended. Refrigerate until ready to serve.

Per serving: 28 calories, 0 g fat (0 g sat fat), 3 g protein, 6 g carbohydrate, 0 g fiber, 1 mg cholesterol, 180 mg sodium

Tahini Dip

Tahini, a Mediterranean staple, is a paste made from sesame seeds. It's a great source of calcium and healthful monounsaturated oils.

SERVES 1

2 teaspoons tahini
1 tablespoon lemon juice
1 tablespoon water
Pinch of garlic powder
Pinch of salt

In a small bowl, stir together the tahini, lemon juice, water, garlic powder, and salt until blended. Refrigerate until ready to serve.

Per serving: 64 calories, 5 g fat (<1 g sat fat), 2 g protein, 4 g carbohydrate, <1 g fiber, 0 mg cholesterol, 150 mg sodium

Spinach Yogurt Dip

Spinach is on every nutritionist's short list of superstar foods. It's an exceptional source of fiber, vitamin A, vitamin K, potassium, magnesium, vitamin C, and calcium.

SERVES 1

$1/2$ cup baby spinach

$1/4$ cup fat-free plain yogurt

Pinch of garlic powder

1 teaspoon finely grated Parmesan cheese

1. Grind the spinach in a small food processor.

2. In a small bowl, stir together the spinach, yogurt, garlic powder, and cheese until blended. Refrigerate until ready to serve.

Per serving: 38 calories, <1 g fat (0 g sat fat), 3 g protein, 6 g carbohydrate, <1 g fiber, 3 mg cholesterol, 84 mg sodium

Sweet Cinnamon Yogurt Dip

Cinnamon provides a concentrated dose of antioxidants, along with calcium, potassium, fiber, and iron. But hey—we're only interested in its great taste!

SERVES 1

$1/2$ cup fat-free plain yogurt

1 teaspoon natural honey

Pinch of ground cinnamon

In a small bowl, stir together the yogurt, honey, and cinnamon until blended. Refrigerate until ready to serve.

Per serving: 72 calories, 0 g fat (0 g sat fat), 5 g protein, 15 g carbohydrate, 0 g fiber, 3 mg cholesterol, 68 mg sodium

Thyme Yogurt Dip

Thyme is a rich source of calcium, iron, magnesium, and potassium and a good source of antioxidants and vitamin K. Its slightly "salty" spiciness can be helpful in reducing sodium intake.

SERVES 1

¼ cup fat-free plain yogurt
1 teaspoon fresh thyme or ¼ teaspoon dried
Pinch of garlic powder
Pinch of salt

In a small bowl, stir together the yogurt, thyme, garlic powder, and salt until blended. Refrigerate until ready to serve.

Per serving: 27 calories, 0 g fat (0 g sat fat), 3 g protein, 5 g carbohydrate, 0 g fiber, 1 mg cholesterol, 189 mg sodium

Satisfaction at the Flavor Point

THE FLAVOR FACTS

Name: Ron Steeves

Age: 55

Hometown: Ansonia, Connecticut

Family status: Married with three adult children, ages 29, 30, and 31

Occupation: Locksmith

Starting weight: 237

Pounds lost: 21 in 12 weeks

Health stats: Blood pressure dropped 16 points; waist measurement shrank $2\frac{1}{2}$ inches

---

"I went on the program simply because I needed to lose weight—I was about 40 pounds overweight when I started. My old habits weren't good. I didn't eat breakfast. I would have coffee at 6:30 A.M. and then go until noon without eating. Then I'd eat a meal, like a potpie, for lunch and not eat again until dinner—and I'd eat a big dinner.

Before starting the Flavor Point Diet, I never was able to stick with a diet and lose weight. I thought the theory about the flavor themes and how they work in the brain to control hunger sounded interesting. I thought, 'This just might work.'

"It did, which is especially impressive because I went on vacation twice during my 12 weeks. I've been on diets before, but I've never been reeducated like this. I lost 21 pounds, and I'm thrilled. My wife has been doing it with me, and she's lost about 10 pounds.

"Overall, my tastes have definitely changed. I like more nutritious foods, and I have adopted better habits. I've cut way back on processed bread. I've also gotten away from all the juices and sodas; I drink a lot of water or iced tea instead. I've also stopped eating highly processed potatoes, fries, pasta, and doughnuts.

"For breakfast, I usually choose one of the plan's flavor-friendly options and eat cereal. I was never a big breakfast person, and I can just eat the cereal quickly and go. For lunch, I usually have a salad. The cafeteria where I work serves some awesome salads with chicken, tuna, or egg, so I grab one of those. Later in the afternoon, I'll have some fruit, and that carries me through to dinner.

"Snack-wise, I love the carrots. If I'm looking for a snack when I get home from work, I'll throw a bunch of baby carrots on a dish and take them outside with me—I just love them. If I want something sweet, I now walk through the kitchen and grab a banana or an orange instead of a brownie.

"Speaking of brownies and desserts, although they looked really good, my wife and I have chosen not to make the desserts on the program. I knew if I kept the sweets around, my craving for sweets wouldn't go away. I grew up in a household where we had pie or cake after dinner every night, so I knew if I did away with sweets altogether, I'd lose weight faster.

"I've also been doing a lot of walking. Even while on vacation, I walked about 2 to 3 miles a day, which has helped to speed up my weight loss.

"I found the program very flexible. When I was on a cruise a few weeks ago, I had fresh fruit in the morning and then a salad for lunch. At dinner, I ate what they served, but I had one serving, and that was it.

"The flavor themes were a unique aspect of Dr. Katz's program, and they worked. My favorites were the tomato day and most of the nut days. I also loved the recipes that included strawberries.

"People have noticed my weight loss and told me I look great. I've really noticed the loss in my stomach—my waistline is shrinking, which is a really good thing. I'm going to stick with it. I plan to lose the other 20 pounds within the next few months—and, with the help of this program, keep those pounds off for life." ■

LUNCHES

Almond, Green Bean, and Quinoa Salad

To save time when preparing this delicious recipe, cook the quinoa ahead of time and refrigerate it to use on a regular basis. You can substitute bulgur wheat for the quinoa if you like.

SERVES 1

1½ cups frozen French-cut green beans
1   teaspoon Dijon mustard
2   teaspoons balsamic vinegar
2   teaspoons extra-virgin olive oil
    Pinch of salt
    Freshly ground black pepper to taste
½   cup cooked quinoa
1   teaspoon crumbled feta cheese
½   red onion, thinly sliced
2   tablespoons chopped almonds

1. Bring 2 cups of water to a boil in a medium saucepan. Add the green beans and cook for 2 minutes (do not overcook). Drain and set aside.

2. In a large bowl, whisk the mustard, vinegar, oil, salt, and pepper. Add the green beans and toss to coat.

3. Add the quinoa, cheese, onion, and almonds and toss to combine.

Per serving: 363 calories, 18 g fat (2 g sat fat), 12 g protein, 43 g carbohydrate, 12 g fiber, 1 mg cholesterol, 398 mg sodium

Apple, Fennel, Walnut, and Barley Salad

The combination of tart apple and cooked barley creates a perfect blend.
Cook the barley ahead of time and refrigerate it so you can have this lunch ready
in the time it takes to chop the apple and fennel. If you like, you can substitute
wheat berries for the barley.

SERVES 1

$\frac{1}{3}$ cup hulled barley

1 apple, rinsed, cored, and chopped

1 bulb fennel, rinsed, trimmed, and thinly sliced

1 tablespoon chopped walnuts

2 tablespoons Newman's Own Light Italian Dressing

Fresh arugula leaves, rinsed and patted dry

1. Bring $1\frac{1}{2}$ cups water to a boil in a medium saucepan. Add the barley and cook for 15 minutes. Drain in a colander and rinse with cold water.

2. In a medium bowl, combine the barley, apple, fennel, walnuts, and dressing. Mix well and serve over the arugula.

Per serving: 358 calories, 13 g fat (2 sat fat), 7 g protein, 60 g carbohydrate, 16 g fiber,
0 mg cholesterol, 388 mg sodium

Coconut Shrimp and Avocado Salad

Our family loves this nutritious tropical delight!

SERVES 1

6   frozen medium easy-peel shrimp

1   teaspoon extra-virgin olive oil

½   avocado, peeled and sliced

Juice of 2 limes (about 3 tablespoons)

2   tablespoons light unsweetened coconut milk

1   scallion, diced

Pinch of salt

Chopped fresh cilantro to taste

1. Quickly thaw the shrimp by rinsing in cold water. Peel and pat dry.

2. Heat the oil in a cast-iron grill pan over high heat. When the oil is very hot, add the shrimp and grill for 2 to 3 minutes on each side (do not overcook).

3. Place the shrimp and avocado in a salad bowl or on a salad plate.

4. In a small bowl, combine the lime juice, coconut milk, scallion, salt, and cilantro.

Pour over the shrimp and avocado and stir gently to blend.

Per serving: 285 calories, 22 g fat (5 g sat fat), 10 g protein, 17 g carbohydrate, 6 g fiber, 55 mg cholesterol, 231 mg sodium

Black Bean, Corn, and Tomato Salad

If you have time to open a can, you have time to throw this complete lunch together in a flash!

SERVES 1

1/2 cup canned black beans, rinsed and drained

1/2 cup canned or frozen corn, rinsed and drained

1 medium tomato, sliced

2 cups loosely packed baby spinach

2 teaspoons extra-virgin olive oil

2 teaspoons balsamic vinegar

1/8 teaspoon ground cumin

   Pinch of salt*

   Freshly ground black pepper to taste

In a medium bowl, combine the beans, corn, tomato, spinach, oil, vinegar, and cumin. Toss well and season with the salt and pepper.

Per serving: 257 calories, 10 g fat (1 g sat fat), 10 g protein, 34 g carbohydrate, 12 g fiber, 0 mg cholesterol, 588 mg sodium

*You don't need to use much, if any, salt in this dish because the residual sodium in the canned beans and corn adds flavor.

Fresh Mint Salade Niçoise

The fresh mint adds a refreshing touch to this classic salad.

SERVES 1

- ½ teaspoon Dijon mustard
- 2 teaspoons extra-virgin olive oil
- 2 teaspoons vinegar
- Pinch of salt
- Freshly ground black pepper to taste
- ½ head Boston lettuce, rinsed and drained
- 2 ounces water-packed tuna, drained
- 1 hard-cooked egg, sliced
- ½ tomato, sliced
- 2 tablespoons chopped fresh mint

1. In a small bowl, whisk the mustard, olive oil, vinegar, salt, and pepper.

2. Place the lettuce in a salad bowl or on a salad plate and top with the tuna, egg, tomato, and mint. Pour on the dressing.

Per serving: 242 calories, 14 g fat (3 g sat fat), 21 g protein, 5 g carbohydrate, 1 g fiber, 197 mg cholesterol, 453 mg sodium

Lemon Tabbouleh Salad

A delicious classic salad bursting with lemon flavor, tabbouleh is made with bulgur wheat, a form of steam-cooked, dried, cracked wheat that's an excellent source of fiber.

SERVES 1

$^3/_4$ cup cooked bulgur wheat (page 228)
1 medium tomato, chopped
2 scallions, chopped
   Juice of 1 lemon
1 teaspoon extra-virgin olive oil
   Pinch of onion powder
   Pinch of garlic powder
   Pinch of salt
1 tablespoon chopped fresh mint or 1 teaspoon dried
1 cup mixed greens

In a medium bowl, combine the bulgur, tomato, scallions, lemon juice, oil, onion powder, garlic powder, salt, and mint. Refrigerate until ready to serve over the greens.

Per serving: 222 calories, 6 g fat (<1 g sat fat), 7 g protein, 41 g carbohydrate, 10 g fiber, 0 mg cholesterol, 333 mg sodium

Currant-Lentil Spinach Salad with Feta and Walnuts

Cook the lentils ahead of time and refrigerate them so you can assemble this salad at the last minute. The amounts of cheese and dressing in this recipe are just enough to provide rich taste without endangering your waistline, so don't cheat! Use the variations to adapt it to the flavor theme of the day.

SERVES 1

2 cups baby spinach (prewashed)
1/3 cup cooked lentils (page 229), well drained
1 teaspoon Dijon mustard
2 teaspoons vinegar
2 teaspoons extra-virgin olive oil
1 tablespoon water
   Pinch of salt
   Freshly ground black pepper to taste
1 tablespoon chopped walnuts
2 tablespoons dried currants or raisins
2 teaspoons feta cheese, crumbled

1. In a medium bowl, combine the spinach and lentils.

2. In a small bowl, stir together the mustard, vinegar, oil, water, salt, and pepper.

3. Add the dressing to the spinach mixture and toss to combine. Sprinkle with the nuts, currants, and cheese.

Per serving: 293 calories, 16 g fat (3 g sat fat), 10 g protein, 32 g carbohydrate, 9 g fiber, 6 mg cholesterol, 343 mg sodium

VARIATIONS

Cranberry-Lentil Mixed Greens Salad with Feta and Pecans:
Replace the spinach with mixed greens. Replace the walnuts with

pecans and add 1 tablespoon dried cranberries instead of the currants in step 3.

Per serving: 301 calories, 17 g fat (3 g sat fat), 10 g protein, 31 g carbohydrate, 9 g fiber, 6 mg cholesterol, 381 mg sodium

Curry, Lentil, and Spinach Salad with Gorgonzola and Walnuts:
Add $1/8$ teaspoon mild curry powder to the dressing in step 2. Omit the currants and replace the feta with Gorgonzola in step 3.

Per serving: 254 calories, 16 g fat (3 g sat fat), 10 g protein, 20 g carbohydrate, 8 g fiber, 4 mg cholesterol, 424 mg sodium

Orange-Lentil Spinach Salad with Feta and Pecans: Use the juice of $1/2$ orange (about $1/4$ cup) instead of the water. Replace the walnuts with pecans and omit the currants.

Per serving: 278 calories, 16 g fat (2 g sat fat), 9 g protein, 28 g carbohydrate, 8 g fiber, 2 mg cholesterol, 452 mg sodium

Pecan, Lentil, and Tomato Mixed Greens Salad: Replace the spinach with mixed greens. Replace the walnuts with pecans and add $1/2$ sliced tomato instead of the cheese in step 3.

Per serving: 263 calories, 16 g fat (2 g sat fat), 10 g protein, 25 g carbohydrate, 10 g fiber, 0 mg cholesterol, 399 mg sodium

Peanut-Cucumber Salad

Peanuts provide a good amount of healthful polyunsaturated and monounsaturated oils, as well as magnesium and vitamin E. Cucumbers are exceptionally low in calories and a good source of beta-carotene and potassium.

SERVES 1

2   cucumbers, seeded and thinly sliced into half-moons
$1/2$ small red onion, thinly sliced
2   tablespoons rice wine vinegar or red wine vinegar
2   tablespoons chopped dry-roasted unsalted peanuts
$1/4$ teaspoon red-pepper flakes
Pinch of salt
1   whole wheat pita*

In a medium bowl, stir together the cucumbers, onion, vinegar, peanuts, pepper flakes, and salt. Refrigerate until ready to serve with the pita.

Per serving: 332 calories, 10 g fat (1 g sat fat), 15 g protein, 50 g carbohydrate, 12 g fiber, 0 mg cholesterol, 389 mg sodium

*See the appendix for recommended brands.

Red Onion, White Bean, Lentil, and Tomato Salad

This salad is perfect for a summer picnic—even one in your kitchen—and provides a wonderful combination of nutrients. Onion and tomato are rich sources of antioxidants, while beans and lentils provide protein and soluble fiber.

SERVES 1

$\frac{1}{3}$ cup canned white cannellini beans, rinsed and drained

$\frac{1}{3}$ cup cooked lentils (page 229)

1 medium tomato, chopped

$\frac{1}{2}$ red onion, thinly sliced

2 teaspoons extra-virgin olive oil

2 teaspoons red wine vinegar

Pinch of salt

Freshly ground black pepper to taste

In a medium bowl, combine the beans, lentils, tomato, onion, oil, vinegar, salt, and pepper. Refrigerate until ready to serve.

Per serving: 349 calories, 13 g fat (1 g sat fat), 12 g protein, 46 g carbohydrate, 12 g fiber, 0 mg cholesterol, 403 mg sodium

Spinach and Turkey Chef's Salad

*Unlike most chef's salads, this one omits processed deli meats, cheeses, and crou-
tons, which all contain salt, sugar, and saturated fat. This healthful version delivers
great taste along with great nutrition.*

SERVES 1

2 teaspoons extra-virgin olive oil

1 teaspoon Dijon mustard

1 tablespoon balsamic vinegar

  Pinch of salt

  Freshly ground black pepper to taste

2 cups baby spinach

1 tomato, sliced

3 slices roast turkey, cut into strips*

1. In a small bowl, combine the oil, mustard, vinegar, salt, and pepper.

2. Place the spinach in a salad bowl or on a salad plate and top with the
   tomato and turkey. Pour on the dressing.

Per serving: 240 calories, 11 g fat (1 g sat fat), 19 g protein, 16 g carbohydrate, 4 g fiber,
37 mg cholesterol, 573 mg sodium

*Choose turkey with no added fat, sugar, or water, such as Plainville brand.

Tomato and Black Bean Mediterranean Salad

Easy, quick, and very filling!

SERVES 1

¹/₂ cup canned black beans, rinsed and drained

1 medium fresh tomato, chopped

2 teaspoons extra-virgin olive oil

1 teaspoon balsamic vinegar

2 teaspoons feta cheese

   Freshly ground black pepper to taste

¹/₂ whole wheat pita*

In a medium bowl, stir together the beans, tomato, oil, vinegar, feta, and pepper. Stuff the filling into the pita.

Per serving: 334 calories, 12 g fat (3 g sat fat), 13 g protein, 46 g carbohydrate, 12 g fiber, 6 mg cholesterol, 256 mg sodium

*See the appendix for recommended brands.

Stuffed Tomato with Thyme Tuna Salad

The ground Kashi crackers in this tuna salad create the perfect consistency and provide plenty of fiber and flavor.

SERVES 1

5   Kashi TLC Original 7-Grain Crackers
1   large tomato
3   ounces water-packed tuna, drained
1   teaspoon Dijon mustard
1¹/₂ tablespoons fat-free plain yogurt
    Chopped celery to taste
1   teaspoon fresh thyme or ¹/₄ teaspoon dried
    Pinch of salt

1. Grind the crackers in a coffee grinder or small food processor or crush them with your fingers. Cut the tomato in half and core it.

2. In a medium bowl, combine the tuna, mustard, yogurt, crackers, celery, thyme, and salt to blend. Stuff both halves of the tomato with the tuna salad.

Per serving: 189 calories, 2 g fat (0 g sat fat), 25 g protein, 17 g carbohydrate, 3 g fiber, 26 mg cholesterol, 615 mg sodium

Portobello Mushroom, Gorgonzola, and Sun-Dried Tomato Sandwich

The Gorgonzola cheese does make this sandwich a bit indulgent, but like everything else at the Flavor Point, the overall nutrition is top-notch. If it also happens to taste sinfully delicious, don't worry—you don't need to feel guilty!

SERVES 1

2 portobello mushrooms, sliced*

2 slices whole grain bread

1 tablespoon oil-packed julienned sun-dried tomatoes, drained

1 tablespoon Gorgonzola cheese

Alfalfa sprouts to taste

1. Coat a cast-iron grill pan with olive oil spray. Add the mushrooms and cook over high heat for a few minutes on each side until tender.

2. Place the mushrooms on 1 slice of bread, top with the tomatoes, cheese, and sprouts, and add the second slice of bread.

Per serving: 236 calories, 5 g fat (2 g sat fat), 11 g protein, 41 g carbohydrate, 14 g fiber, 6 mg cholesterol, 327 mg sodium

*Look for packaged presliced mushrooms.

Walnut Chicken Salad

Cook the chicken ahead and refrigerate it to save time when you assemble this delicious salad, or use 3 ounces of drained water-packed chicken. Use the variations of this recipe to adapt it to the flavor theme of the day.

SERVES 1

$\frac{1}{2}$ teaspoon salt + pinch of salt

1   3-ounce chicken cutlet

1   tablespoon chopped walnuts

2   teaspoons fat-free plain yogurt

1   teaspoon Dijon mustard

1   teaspoon extra-virgin olive oil

$\frac{1}{2}$ teaspoon apple cider vinegar

   Pinch of garlic powder

   Freshly ground black pepper to taste

1. Bring $1\frac{1}{2}$ cups water to a simmer in a medium saucepan and add salt. Add the chicken and cook for 10 minutes, or until cooked through. Alternatively, grill it in a cast-iron grill pan coated with olive oil spray. Let cool and finely chop.

2. In a small bowl, combine the chicken, walnuts, yogurt, mustard, oil, vinegar, garlic powder, salt, and pepper. Refrigerate until ready to serve.

Per serving: 243 calories, 13 g fat (2 g sat fat), 28 g protein, 4 g carbohydrate, 1 g fiber, 73 mg cholesterol, 314 mg sodium

VARIATIONS

Apple-Walnut Chicken Salad: Add $\frac{1}{2}$ tart green apple, finely chopped.

Per serving: 273 calories, 13 g fat (2 g sat fat), 28 g protein, 12 g carbohydrate, 2 g fiber, 73 mg cholesterol, 169 mg sodium

THE FLAVOR POINT DIET RECIPES   177

Pineapple-Walnut Chicken Salad: Add 1 tablespoon drained canned unsweetened crushed pineapple.

Per serving: 253 calories, 13 g fat (2 g sat fat), 28 g protein, 6 g carbohydrate, 1 g fiber, 73 mg cholesterol, 325 mg sodium

Dill Chicken Salad Sandwich

This isn't your mother's chicken salad! Our version steers clear of mayonnaise and adds whole grain goodness and fiber with Kashi crackers, but still delivers great taste. Judge for yourself!

SERVES 1

5   Kashi TLC Original 7-Grain Crackers

3   ounces water-packed chicken, drained

1   teaspoon Dijon mustard

1½ tablespoons plain fat-free yogurt

    Chopped celery to taste

1   teaspoon fresh dill or ⅛ teaspoon dried

½   tomato, sliced

    Lettuce

2   slices whole grain bread or 2 pieces whole grain melba toast*

1. Grind the crackers in a coffee grinder or small food processor or crush them with your fingers.

2. In a medium bowl, combine the chicken, mustard, yogurt, cracker crumbs, celery, and dill.

3. Spread between bread, or serve with melba toast.

Per serving: 298 calories, 5 g fat (2 g sat fat), 23 g protein, 43 g carbohydrate, 13 g fiber, 52 mg cholesterol, 669 mg sodium

*See the appendix for recommended brands.

Pumpkin and Chocolate Grilled Panini

This probably isn't a recipe you would have come up with on your own! It's unusual, we admit, but give it a try. We're pretty sure you'll love it (our test subjects did!). Both pumpkin and chocolate are rich in antioxidant nutrients and fiber.

SERVES 1

1   teaspoon Smart Balance spread
2   slices whole grain bread
2   tablespoons canned pumpkin (no added salt or sugar)
16   Ghirardelli Double Chocolate Chips
1   tablespoon chopped pecans

1. Spread ½ teaspoon of the spread on 1 side of each slice of bread.

2. Spread the pumpkin on the plain side of 1 slice, line up the chocolate chips in 4 rows of 4, and sprinkle with the nuts. Place the second slice on top with the spread facing up.

3. Place the sandwich in a hot panini grill or a nonstick skillet over medium heat, close the grill (if using a skillet, press the sandwich with a spatula), and grill for 2 to 3 minutes (if using a skillet, turn the sandwich and press again).

Per serving: 261 calories, 12 g fat (3 g sat fat), 6 g protein, 38 g carbohydrate, 12 g fiber, 0 mg cholesterol, 192 mg sodium

VARIATION

Chocolate and Banana Grilled Panini: Use ½ sliced banana instead of the pumpkin and omit the pecans.

Per serving: 258 calories, 7 g fat (3 g sat fat), 6 g protein, 51 g carbohydrate, 12 g fiber, 0 mg cholesterol, 176 mg sodium

DINNERS

Sesame-Soy Chicken Cutlets

If you use the thin cutlets, this dinner is ready in less than 15 minutes.

SERVES 4

4 chicken cutlets (about 1½ pounds)
Pinch of salt
2 teaspoons extra-virgin olive oil
2 teaspoons grated fresh ginger or garlic
3 tablespoons sesame seeds, toasted
¼ cup low-sodium soy sauce
¼ cup sherry

1. Rinse the chicken and pat dry. Salt lightly (use no more than ⅛ teaspoon) and set aside.

2. Heat the oil in a nonstick skillet. Add the ginger and sauté for a few seconds.

3. Add the chicken and cook for 4 to 5 minutes. Turn the chicken, add the sesame seeds, soy sauce, and sherry, and cook for 4 to 5 minutes (do not overcook).

Per serving: 275 calories, 11 g fat (2 g sat fat), 36 g protein, 5 g carbohydrate, 1 g fiber, 94 mg cholesterol, 706 mg sodium

Carrot Cider–Glazed Chicken

No one (besides the chef) can ever figure out the secret ingredient in this dish. It's carrot juice, of course, but you don't need to tell! The subtle sweetness of the carrot juice helps you reach the Flavor Point quickly and makes this glaze a favorite for grownups and kids alike. Enjoy it to your heart's content—literally!

SERVES 4

4 chicken thighs, skin removed
4 chicken drumsticks, skin removed
$3/4$ teaspoon salt
$1/4$ cup Arrowhead Mills Organic Pastry Flour*
$2 1/2$ teaspoons extra-virgin olive oil
1 teaspoon minced fresh ginger
2 whole cloves garlic, thickly sliced
$1/2$ cup carrot juice
$1/3$ cup apple cider
$1/2$ cup dark beer
1 teaspoon ground coriander[†]

1. Preheat the oven to 375°F. Rinse the chicken and pat dry. Salt lightly (use no more than $1/8$ teaspoon of the salt).

2. Place the flour on a flat plate and dredge the chicken pieces, coating both sides.

3. Drizzle 2 teaspoons of the oil into a large nonstick skillet (it needs to be deep enough to hold 2 cups of liquid) over medium-high heat and sauté the chicken on both sides for 4 to 5 minutes, or until slightly browned. (You'll be tempted to add more oil here, but don't. That's all it needs, really!) Transfer the chicken to a baking pan and set aside.

4. Drizzle the remaining $1/2$ teaspoon oil into the skillet and sauté the ginger for a few seconds. Add the garlic, carrot juice, cider, beer, coriander, and the

remaining salt to the skillet and bring to a boil. Reduce the heat and simmer for 2 to 3 minutes. Pour the liquid over the chicken.

5. Bake for 30 minutes. Turn the pieces and bake for an additional 15 to 20 minutes, or until the chicken almost falls off the bone and the sauce is thick and golden.

Per serving: 271 calories, 11 g fat (3 g sat fat), 27 g protein, 11 g carbohydrate, 1 g fiber, 90 mg cholesterol, 543 mg sodium

*You can also use Hodgson Mill Oat Bran Flour.

†For maximum flavor, grind whole coriander freshly in a coffee grinder.

Chicken with Chocolate Port Wine Sauce

Remember the mouthwatering scene in the movie Chocolat *where everyone gathers around a feast of dishes imbued with chocolate flavor? This luscious sauce could well have been in that scene. It's rich and enticing, with just a hint of bittersweet chocolate—just enough to make the sauce creamy and velvety (velouté). This recipe is time-consuming but well worth it if you want to indulge in a chocolate day!*

SERVES 4

SAUCE

1   tablespoon slivered almonds

2   medium shallots

3   cloves garlic

2   teaspoons extra-virgin olive oil

1   can (15 ounces) diced tomatoes, drained

½   teaspoon salt

   Freshly ground black pepper to taste

1   cup fat-free chicken broth

1   cup port wine

1   ounce Ghirardelli bittersweet chocolate

2   teaspoons pink peppercorns

1   teaspoon cognac

CHICKEN

4   whole skinless chicken breasts (about 2 pounds), halved

   Pinch of salt

   Freshly ground black pepper to taste

1. **To make the sauce:** Grind the almonds to a fine powder in a coffee grinder. Grind the shallots and garlic in a small food processor.

2. Heat the oil in a heavy skillet and lightly sauté the almonds, shallots, and garlic for 2 to 3 minutes.

3. Add the tomatoes, salt, and pepper and cook for 5 to 6 minutes. Add the broth and wine and bring to a boil.

4. Reduce the heat and add the chocolate, stirring constantly to blend. Simmer for 15 minutes. Remove from the heat, cover, and let stand for a few minutes.

5. Ladle the mixture into a blender and process until smooth. Strain through a medium sieve into a small saucepan and reserve the liquid, discarding what remains in the sieve.

6. *To make the chicken:* Rinse the chicken and pat dry. Season both sides lightly with the salt and pepper.

7. Coat a large cast-iron grill pan with olive oil spray and heat over medium-high heat. Add the chicken and grill on each side for 8 to 10 minutes, or until cooked through.

8. Return the saucepan to the stove and rub the peppercorns between your palms to crush them into the sauce. Add the cognac and simmer just until heated through. Serve over the chicken.

Per serving: 403 calories, 11 g fat (3 g sat fat), 41 g protein, 19 g carbohydrate, 1 g fiber, 102 mg cholesterol, 865 mg sodium

Chicken in Creamy Dijon Mushroom Sauce

Your family will never suspect that this wonderful, rich and creamy dish has no added fat. There's no need to add salt since there's enough in the mustard, broth, and buttermilk to provide flavor. If you're lucky enough to have leftovers, use them to make a great sandwich for tomorrow's lunch.

SERVES 4

1¼ pounds chicken cutlets or tenderloins

3 tablespoons Dijon mustard

¼ cup fat-free plain yogurt

¼ cup fat-free chicken broth

½ cup vermouth

1 teaspoon extra-virgin olive oil

1 package (8 ounces) sliced mushrooms (about 3 cups), washed and drained

¼ cup fat-free buttermilk

1 tablespoon whole grain mustard

Freshly ground black pepper to taste

1. Preheat the oven to 375°F. Rinse the chicken and pat dry.

2. In a small bowl, combine the Dijon mustard and yogurt. Coat the chicken with the mixture, then cover and refrigerate for at least 15 minutes (this can be done the night before; the chicken will be more tender, and you can assemble the dish quickly).

3. Arrange the chicken in a shallow baking dish that can also be used on the stove. In a measuring cup, combine the broth and ¼ cup of the vermouth and pour around the chicken. Bake for about 10 minutes. Turn the chicken once and bake for 10 to 15 minutes, or just until tender (do not overcook).

4. Meanwhile, heat the oil in a nonstick skillet over medium heat. Add the mushrooms and sauté until tender. Drain in a colander and set aside.

5. Transfer the chicken to a plate. Place the baking dish over medium-high heat and add the mushrooms. Bring to a boil and whisk in the buttermilk, whole grain mustard, pepper, and the remaining $\frac{1}{4}$ cup vermouth. Reduce the heat and cook for a few minutes, stirring constantly, until well blended and creamy.

6. Return the chicken to the baking dish and spoon the sauce over it.

Per serving: 242 calories, 5 g fat (1 g sat fat), 32 g protein, 9 g carbohydrate, 1 g fiber, 79 mg cholesterol, 334 mg sodium

Coconut Thai Chicken

Because coconut is relatively high in saturated fat, the Flavor Point Diet uses it spar-ingly. It sure makes for wonderful, slightly exotic flavor, so enjoy!

SERVES 4*

1¼ pounds boneless, skinless chicken breast

¾ teaspoon salt

½ cup hot green tea

¼ cup light unsweetened coconut milk

¼ cup natural peanut butter (no added salt, sugar, or oils)

Juice of 2 limes (about 3 tablespoons)

1 tablespoon grated fresh ginger

1 tablespoon natural honey

2 tablespoons low-sodium soy sauce

Chopped fresh cilantro to taste

2 teaspoons extra-virgin olive oil

1. Rinse the chicken and pat dry. Salt lightly (use no more than ⅛ teaspoon of the salt) and cut into 12 equal pieces. Place in a baking dish.

2. In a blender, combine the tea, coconut milk, peanut butter, lime juice, ginger, honey, soy sauce, cilantro, and the remaining salt. Process until smooth.

3. Pour half of the marinade over the chicken and mix to coat well (you can make the marinade ahead of time and refrigerate for more flavor). Reserve the remaining marinade.

4. Heat the oil in a cast-iron grill pan. When the pan is very hot, add the chicken pieces one by one and grill for 4 to 5 minutes on each side (do not overcook).

5. Transfer the chicken to a serving platter and pour the remaining sauce over it.

Per serving: 308 calories, 14 g fat (3 g sat fat), 33 g protein, 11 g carbohydrate, 1 g fiber, 78 mg cholesterol, 848 mg sodium

*Serving size: 3 pieces

Pistachio-Crusted Chicken

Because chicken cutlets are thin, they cook quickly. This dish is deliciously crunchy on the outside and filled with pistachio flavor!

SERVES 4

12 Kashi TLC Original 7-Grain Crackers
$\frac{1}{2}$ cup roasted salted pistachio nuts
4 chicken cutlets (4 ounces each)
    Pinch of salt
2 teaspoons extra-virgin olive oil

1. Grind the crackers and pistachios in a coffee grinder or small food processor and place in a shallow bowl.

2. Rinse the chicken and pat dry. Salt lightly (use no more than $\frac{1}{8}$ teaspoon).

3. Dredge the chicken in the crumbs, coating both sides.

4. Heat the oil in a large nonstick skillet. Add the chicken and sear on each side for 4 to 5 minutes.

Per serving: 260 calories, 13 g fat (2 g sat fat), 27 g protein, 9 g carbohydrate, 2 g fiber, 63 mg cholesterol, 232 mg sodium

Roast Chicken with Currant Wine Glaze and Caramelized Onions

This dish always gets high praise. The blend of currants and wine is deliciously sweet. It's quick and easy to prepare, but you need to schedule the time to roast the chicken for about an hour so it's glazed to perfection.

SERVES 4

- 1 medium roasting chicken
- $\frac{1}{4}$ teaspoon salt
  Freshly ground black pepper to taste
- 2 teaspoons extra-virgin olive oil
- 2 yellow onions, thinly sliced
- 1 cup red wine
- 1 cup fat-free chicken broth
- 6 tablespoons dried currants
- 2 tablespoons rinsed and drained capers
- 2 teaspoons crushed dried rosemary

1. Preheat the oven to 375°F. Rinse the chicken and pat dry. Remove all of the bottom skin and as much of the skin on the sides as you can with kitchen scissors, leaving only the skin on top. Lightly salt and pepper the cavity and place the chicken in a roasting pan.

2. Heat the oil in a heavy skillet. Add the onions and cook for about 5 minutes, or until soft. (Do not add more oil; the onions will "sweat" perfectly with this amount and don't need to brown at this point. They will caramelize in the oven.)

3. Add the wine, broth, currants, capers, and rosemary, bring to a boil, and simmer for 5 to 7 minutes.

4. Pour the liquid over the chicken and bake for 1 hour, or until the sauce thickens and becomes a glaze.

Per serving: 395 calories, 9 g fat (2 g sat fat), 51 g protein, 22 g carbohydrate, 2 g fiber, 155 mg cholesterol, 857 mg sodium

Grilled Chicken with Caramelized Onion on Pita

This tasty, fun dinner can get messy! Don't even try to stuff it into the pita, or the pita will break apart.

SERVES 4

1¼ pounds boneless, skinless chicken breasts
¼ teaspoon salt
2 tablespoons extra-virgin olive oil
2 yellow onions, thinly sliced
½ cup oil-packed sun-dried tomatoes, drained
   Freshly ground black pepper to taste
4 large whole wheat pitas*
   Mixed greens

1. Rinse the chicken and pat dry. Salt lightly (use no more than ⅛ teaspoon of the salt).

2. Heat the oil in a medium nonstick skillet over medium-high heat. Add the onions and the remaining salt. Reduce the heat, cover, and cook, stirring occasionally, for 10 minutes.

3. Add the tomatoes and cook for 10 more minutes, or until the onions are soft and golden.

4. Meanwhile, coat a large cast-iron grill pan with olive oil spray and heat over medium-high heat. Grill the chicken on each side for 6 to 8 minutes and add the pepper. While the chicken is hot, cut into strips with a sharp knife.

5. To serve, place a pita flat on each of 4 plates and top with equal portions of the greens, chicken, and onion mixture.

Per serving: 413 calories, 14 g fat (2 g sat fat), 36 g protein, 38 g carbohydrate, 7 g fiber, 78 mg cholesterol, 360 mg sodium

*See the appendix for recommended brands.

Grilled Chicken
with White Beans Provençal

If you have the time to open two cans of beans and grill some chicken, you'll have yourself a Chow Now dinner! You just have to be sure to use thin chicken cutlets and have the vermouth on hand in your pantry.

SERVES 4

4   chicken cutlets (4 ounces each)
    Pinch of salt
4   teaspoons extra-virgin olive oil
3   cloves garlic*, thickly sliced
½   cup vermouth
1   cup fat-free chicken broth
2   cans (15 ounces each) cannellini beans, rinsed and drained
2   teaspoons dried thyme
    Freshly ground black pepper to taste

1. Rinse the chicken and pat dry. Salt lightly (use no more than ⅛ teaspoon).

2. Heat 2 teaspoons of the oil in a medium nonstick skillet over medium-high heat. Add the garlic and sauté for a few seconds.

3. Add the vermouth and bring to a boil for 1 to 2 minutes. Add the broth and beans and bring to a boil. Reduce the heat, add the thyme and pepper, and simmer for 10 minutes.

4. Meanwhile, heat the remaining 2 teaspoons oil in a large cast-iron grill pan. When the pan is hot, grill the chicken for 2 to 3 minutes on each side, or until cooked through (do not overcook). Serve the beans over the chicken.

Per serving: 385 calories, 8 g fat (1 g sat fat), 33 g protein, 34 g carbohydrate, 8 g fiber, 63 mg cholesterol, 615 mg sodium

* Use prepeeled garlic to save time.

Honey Curry—Glazed Chicken

This dish takes all of 5 minutes to prepare, but it needs a good hour to bake so the juices simmer down to a rich, thick, golden glaze and coat the chicken perfectly (be sure to use only drumsticks, since only they will remain tender and juicy). It's definitely worth the wait. Serve it hot or cold. Make it in advance, refrigerate, and take along on a picnic. The kids will love it because it's sweet, and it's messy fun to eat with their fingers!

SERVES 4

12 chicken drumsticks, skin removed*
 2 tablespoons Dijon mustard
$\frac{1}{4}$ cup lemon juice
$\frac{1}{4}$ cup natural honey
$\frac{1}{4}$ teaspoon mild curry powder
$\frac{1}{2}$ teaspoon salt

1. Preheat the oven to 375°F. Rinse the chicken and pat dry.

2. In a large bowl, combine the mustard, lemon juice, honey, curry powder, and salt. Add the chicken and stir to coat (you can do this ahead of time and refrigerate, covered, overnight if you like).

3. Bake for 1 hour, turning once and basting occasionally, until the chicken almost falls off the bone and the sauce has thickened to a rich golden glaze.

Per serving: 295 calories, 7 g fat (2 g sat fat), 38 g protein, 18 g carbohydrate, 0 g fiber, 123 mg cholesterol, 514 mg sodium

*Ask the butcher at the supermarket to remove it.

Pecan-Crusted Chicken

The pecan crust on this chicken is out of this world! You finish cooking the chicken breasts in the oven so the nutty crust doesn't burn. If you'd like to cut down on time, use the same amount of cutlets. They're thinner and will cook fast enough for the crust to stay golden.

SERVES 4*

- 2 boneless, skinless chicken breasts (about 1¼ pounds), halved
- ¼ teaspoon salt
- 15 Kashi TLC Original 7-Grain Crackers
- 2 egg whites
- ½ cup finely chopped pecans
- Freshly ground black pepper to taste
- 2 teaspoons extra-virgin olive oil

1. Preheat the oven to 400°F. Rinse the chicken and pat dry. Salt lightly (use no more than ⅛ teaspoon of the salt) and set aside.

2. Grind the crackers in a coffee grinder or small food processor.

3. In a wide, shallow dish, whisk the egg whites with a fork. On a flat plate, combine the cracker crumbs, pecans, pepper, and the remaining salt.

4. One at a time, dip the chicken pieces first in the egg whites and then in the crumbs, coating both sides well.

5. Heat the oil in a large, nonstick, ovenproof skillet. Add the chicken and cook over medium-high heat for 2 to 3 minutes on each side, or until browned. Transfer the pan to the oven for 5 minutes to finish cooking.

Per serving: 291 calories, 16 g fat (2 g sat fat), 27 g protein, 9 g carbohydrate, 2 g fiber, 63 mg cholesterol, 278 mg sodium

*Serving size: ½ breast or 1 cutlet

Mexican Stuffed Bell Peppers

A complete meal stuffed in a pepper!

SERVES 4

  4   red or yellow bell peppers*
  2   teaspoons extra-virgin olive oil
  1   clove garlic, minced
  8   ounces lean ground turkey
  1   can (15 ounces) fat-free refried beans
1¹/₂   cups mild salsa†
 ³/₄   cup cooked bulgur wheat (page 228)
 ¹/₄   cup grated part-skim mozzarella cheese

1. Preheat the oven to 350°F.

2. Rinse and dry the peppers. Slice off the tops, remove the cores and seeds, and place in a baking pan.

3. Heat the oil in a skillet. Add the garlic and sauté for a few seconds. Add the ground turkey and cook, stirring, for 5 minutes.

4. Add the beans, salsa, and cooked bulgur and cook for 3 to 4 minutes, or until bubbly.

5. Stuff each pepper with ¹/₄ of the stuffing and top with ¹/₄ of the cheese. Bake for 20 to 25 minutes, then broil for 5 minutes, or until the cheese is sizzling and golden.

Per serving: 321 calories, 10 g fat (3 g sat fat), 19 g protein, 39 g carbohydrate, 10 g fiber, 51 mg cholesterol, 763 mg sodium

*Pick short, stout ones that will stand upright.

†See the appendix for recommended brands.

Satisfaction at the Flavor Point

THE FLAVOR FACTS

Name: Laura Coppola

Age: 40

Hometown: Ansonia, Connecticut

Family status: Married

Occupation: Buyer for hospital purchasing department

Starting weight: 178

Pounds lost: 19 in 12 weeks

Health stats: Cholesterol dropped 11 points; blood pressure dropped 10 points; waist measurement shrank 4 inches; 6 percent decline in body fat

"Since my father died a few years ago, I ate out of depression and put on a lot of weight. I tried Weight Watchers for a while, and it worked, but I didn't stick to it because it was too much measuring. I was looking for another program, and Dr. Katz's plan came into my life at just the right time.

"Not only was the timing perfect, but Dr. Katz's program is so great—I love the recipes, and I'm learning to shop, cook, and eat healthfully. My energy level is much higher (I can go from 8 in the morning to 11 at night without stopping), my clothes fit much better, and I feel like I can breathe.

"I have to admit, when I took a first glance through the meal plan, there were some recipes that made me say, 'Eww' because the combinations of ingredients were strange. But when you put them all together, they taste really good. You can take a plain old piece of chicken or fish and add poppy seeds or something to it, and it's wonderful. I never would have thought to do those things before.

"My favorite breakfast dishes were the omelets because they were both flavorful and filling; I usually ate them on the weekends when I had more time to cook. During the week, I ate the whole grain cereal for breakfast to save time.

"For lunch, I particularly liked the walnut chicken salad and the tuna salad because they were easy to prepare and tasted excellent. I also liked them because I ate them on whole wheat bread, which was a switch from eating all the salads.

"My favorite dinners were Pan-Seared Tilapia with Lemon Chives and Capers and Shrimp Pasta Primavera with Basil Pesto. The pasta primavera was particularly good, and sometimes I would add grilled chicken breast to it for variety. Even better, my husband—a really finicky eater—has been eating a lot of the meals with me.

"Another great thing about Dr. Katz's program is that I never feel hungry or deprived. If I do start to feel a little hungry, it's not until 9 or 10 o'clock, and I just have one of the snacks. If I feel a craving coming on, like for chocolate, I just make something out of the plan with chocolate in it. (I'm a chocolate lover, so it was great that after the first 3 weeks, the program started to incorporate chocolate.) The chocolate brownies and the oatmeal cookies with chocolate chips are really good.

"It's also really easy to adjust to the program if I eat out. My husband and I pick restaurants that offer healthy choices, or we look for a place with a salad bar.

"The best part of the program is that it works—I look at myself in the mirror and my face looks thinner, I can put on a pair of size 7 or 8 shorts (I used to wear a 14), and people at work tell me I look great.

"I really love Dr. Katz's program; I am definitely going to try to stick to it for life. It's so much better than all the fad diets out there."

Apple-Prune Chicken

This is an absolute delight! The apples and prunes make a perfect pair.

SERVES 4

 4 split chicken breasts (about 2 pounds), skin removed
 $3/4$ teaspoon salt
 $1/4$ cup Arrowhead Mills Organic Pastry Flour*
 3 teaspoons extra-virgin olive oil
 4 cloves garlic, thickly sliced
 1 medium apple, rinsed and sliced
 $1^1/2$ cups 100% apple juice or apple cider
 $1/2$ cup pitted prunes

1. Preheat the oven to 375°F. Rinse the chicken and pat dry. Salt lightly (use no more than $1/8$ teaspoon of the salt).

2. Place the flour on a flat plate and dredge each chicken piece, coating on both sides.

3. Add 2 teaspoons of the oil to a large baking pan over medium-high heat and briefly sauté the chicken on both sides for 4 to 5 minutes, or until slightly browned. (You'll be tempted to add more oil, but don't. That's all it needs, really!) Transfer the chicken to a plate and set aside.

4. Add the remaining 1 teaspoon oil to the pan and sauté the garlic and apple for 1 to 2 minutes.

5. Add the apple juice, prunes, and the remaining salt and bring to a boil. Reduce the heat and simmer for 5 to 8 minutes.

6. Return the chicken to the pan and spoon some of the liquid over it. Bake for 30 minutes. Turn the pieces and bake for an additional 10 to 15 minutes, or until the chicken is tender and the sauce is thick and glistening. If you like, crush the prunes so they become part of the sauce.

Per serving: 328 calories, 7 g fat (1 g sat fat), 30 g protein, 36 g carbohydrate, 3 g fiber, 76 mg cholesterol, 654 mg sodium

*You can also use Hodgson Mill Oat Bran Flour.

Cranberry and Sweet Onion Turkey Cutlets

If you're in the mood for a little taste of Thanksgiving in a flash, this is the recipe for you! It's one of those "throw-everything-in-the-pan" kinds of dishes that's very simple and quick to prepare and very satisfying. It takes a good 20 minutes to simmer.

SERVES 4

4   skinless turkey breast cutlets (1½ pounds)*
    Pinch of salt
1   medium yellow onion, sliced
1   tablespoon extra-virgin olive oil
½   cup fat-free chicken broth
¾   cup 100% cranberry juice
¾   cup dried cranberries
6   dried prunes
1   tablespoon balsamic vinegar
    Freshly ground black pepper to taste

1. Rinse the turkey and pat dry. Salt lightly (use no more than ⅛ teaspoon).

2. In a large skillet over medium heat, sauté the onions in the oil for 3 to 5 minutes.

3. Add the turkey and cook, turning once, for 5 to 8 minutes, or until it begins to brown.

4. Add the broth, cranberry juice, cranberries, prunes, and vinegar and cook for 20 to 25 minutes, or until the turkey is well done and the sauce is rich and thick. Season with the pepper. If you like, crush the prunes in the pan so they become part of the sauce.

Per serving: 351 calories, 5 g fat (<1 g sat fat), 44 g protein, 33 g carbohydrate, 3 g fiber, 105 mg cholesterol, 398 mg sodium

*Look for brands with no added salt or sugar.

Peach-Coriander Turkey
with Oven-Roasted Potatoes and Turnips

The sweet flavor of peach blends wonderfully with the slight tartness of the beer, creating a very satisfying and hearty dinner.

SERVES 4

POTATOES AND TURNIPS

4 small red potatoes, scrubbed and halved

4 turnips, scrubbed, peeled, and cut into large pieces

2 teaspoons extra-virgin olive oil

1 teaspoon garlic powder

1/4 teaspoon salt

Freshly ground black pepper to taste

TURKEY

1 skinless turkey thigh (about 2 pounds), bone in

3/4 teaspoon salt

Freshly ground black pepper to taste

3 tablespoons all-fruit peach jam (no added sugar)*

6 dried peaches

2 tablespoons whole grain mustard

1 tablespoon coriander seeds

3 cloves garlic, minced

1 cup amber imported beer

2 teaspoons extra-virgin olive oil

1. ***To make the potatoes and turnips:*** In a medium bowl, combine the potatoes, turnips, oil, garlic powder, salt, and pepper and toss to coat. Set aside.

2. ***To make the turkey:*** Preheat the oven to 375°F. Coat a baking pan with olive oil spray.

3. Remove the skin from the turkey with kitchen scissors, rinse, and pat dry. Season with salt and pepper (use no more than $\frac{1}{8}$ teaspoon of the salt). Place in the baking pan and set aside.

4. In a small bowl, stir together the jam, peaches, mustard, coriander, garlic, beer, oil, and the remaining salt. Pour over the turkey and bake for 30 to 40 minutes. Add the potatoes and turnips to the pan during the final 20 to 25 minutes of cooking time.

Per serving (turkey): 321 calories, 9 g fat (2 g sat fat), 30 g protein, 26 g carbohydrate, 3 g fiber, 93 mg cholesterol, 664 mg sodium

Per serving (potatoes and turnips): 180 calories, 3 g fat (0 g sat fat), 4 g protein, 35 g carbohydrate, 5 g fiber, 0 mg cholesterol, 238 mg sodium

*See the appendix for recommended brands.

Turkey, Bean, and Thyme Pot au Feu

A pot au feu is one of those feel-good comfort stews that simmer slowly in the oven for a long time and fill the whole house with wonderful smells.

SERVES 4

2 teaspoons extra-virgin olive oil

¾ cup sliced baby carrots

1 medium yellow onion, chopped

4 cloves garlic, thickly sliced

1½ pounds boneless, skinless turkey breast (London broil cut)

2 teaspoons dried thyme

1 bay leaf

Pinch of salt

1 can (15 ounces) diced tomatoes*

2 cups fat-free chicken broth

¾ cup red table wine

2 cans (15 ounces each) small cannellini beans, rinsed and drained

1. Preheat the oven to 350°F.

2. Heat the oil in a large baking pan. Add the carrots, onion, and garlic and sauté for 2 minutes.

3. Add the turkey, thyme, bay leaf, and salt and cook for 8 to 10 minutes. Turn the turkey to brown on the other side.

4. Stir in the tomatoes (with juice), broth, and wine and bring to a boil. Stir in the beans. Transfer to the oven and bake for 1 hour. Remove the bay leaf before serving.

Per serving: 477 calories, 5 g fat (<1 g sat fat), 55 g protein, 44 g carbohydrate, 11 g fiber, 105 mg cholesterol, 857 mg sodium

*See the appendix for recommended brands.

Almond-Crusted Tilapia

This is a great quick and simple dish!

SERVES 4

1$^{1}/_{2}$ pounds tilapia fillets
15   Kashi TLC Original 7-Grain Crackers
2   egg whites
$^{1}/_{2}$ cup finely chopped almonds
$^{1}/_{4}$ teaspoon salt
       Freshly ground black pepper to taste
2   teaspoons extra-virgin olive oil

1. Preheat the oven to 400°F. Rinse the fish, pat dry, and set aside.

2. Grind the crackers in a coffee grinder or small food processor.

3. In a wide, shallow dish, whisk the egg whites with a fork. On a flat plate, combine the crackers, almonds, salt, and pepper.

4. One at a time, dip the fillets first in the egg whites and then in the crumbs, coating both sides well.

5. Heat the oil in a large, nonstick, ovenproof skillet and sear the filets over medium-high heat for 2 to 3 minutes on each side.

6. Transfer the pan to the oven and bake for 5 minutes.

Per serving: 284 calories, 11 g fat (2 g sat fat), 37 g protein, 9 g carbohydrate, 2 g fiber, 83 mg cholesterol, 283 mg sodium

Baked Tilapia with Tomatoes, Olives, and Capers

This is a very tasty way to bake tilapia with a southern French flavor. All the ingredients for this quick and easy dish are mixed right in the baking pan, so you'll have just one pan to clean.

SERVES 4

$1^1/_2$ pounds tilapia fillets
    Pinch of salt
  1 can (15 ounces) diced tomatoes*
  2 tablespoons tomato paste
  2 tablespoons water
$^1/_2$ cup kalamata olives
  2 tablespoons rinsed and drained capers
  2 tablespoons oil-packed sun-dried tomatoes, drained
  1 tablespoon extra-virgin olive oil
  4 cloves garlic, peeled and thickly sliced
  6 cornichons† (optional)
    Freshly ground black pepper to taste

1. Preheat the oven to 375°F.

2. Rinse the fish and pat dry. Salt lightly (use no more than $^1/_8$ teaspoon).

3. In a baking pan, stir together the diced tomatoes (with juice), tomato paste, water, olives, capers, sun-dried tomatoes, oil, garlic, cornichons (if using), and pepper.

4. Add the fish to the baking pan and spoon some of the sauce on top. Bake for 30 minutes, basting once or twice.

Per serving: 292 calories, 10 g fat (2 g sat fat), 34 g protein, 17 g carbohydrate, 3 g fiber, 83 mg cholesterol, 928 mg sodium

*See the appendix for recommended brands.

†These are the baby dill gherkins in the pickle aisle.

Pan-Seared Tilapia with Lemon Chives and Capers

The tender white flesh of this fish is mild and delicious. Even kids love it! It's inexpensive, always found fresh at the supermarket, and cooks very quickly, so it's perfect for Chow Now nights.

SERVES 4

Juice of 2 lemons (about ⅓ cup)

1 tablespoon fresh chives, snipped

1 teaspoon rinsed and drained capers

3 tablespoons extra-virgin olive oil

1½ pounds fresh tilapia fillets

Salt

Freshly ground black pepper to taste

¼ cup Arrowhead Mills Organic Pastry Flour*

1. In a small bowl, stir together the lemon juice, chives, capers, dash of salt, and 2 tablespoons of the oil. Set aside.

2. Rinse the fish and pat dry. Season with the salt (use no more than ⅛ teaspoon) and pepper. Place the flour on a flat plate and dredge the fish, coating both sides.

3. Heat the remaining 1 tablespoon oil in a large nonstick skillet over medium-high heat. Add the fish and cook, turning once, for 7 to 8 minutes, or until tender and browned on both sides.

4. To serve, place a fillet on each of 4 plates and drizzle with the lemon mixture.

Per serving: 261 calories, 12 g fat (2 g sat fat), 33 g protein, 6 g carbohydrate, 1 g fiber, 83 mg cholesterol, 227 mg sodium

*You can also use Hodgson Mill Oat Bran Flour.

Orange Cod

The orange makes this dish very tasty, and it's so quick and easy, you can put it together at the last minute.

SERVES 4

1 tablespoon extra-virgin olive oil

2 tablespoons rice wine vinegar or apple cider vinegar

3 tablespoons frozen 100% orange juice concentrate, thawed

2 tablespoons orange juice

$\frac{1}{2}$ teaspoon salt

Freshly ground black pepper to taste

$1\frac{1}{4}$ pounds codfish (captain's cut)

1 orange, peeled and sliced

1 tablespoon rinsed and drained capers (optional)

Chopped fresh cilantro (optional)

1. Preheat the oven to 400°F.

2. In a medium bowl, stir together the oil, vinegar, orange juice concentrate, orange juice, salt, and pepper. Set aside.

3. Rinse the fish and pat dry. Add to the marinade and turn to coat on both sides. Place in a baking dish and pour the remaining marinade over it.

4. Arrange the orange slices on top of the fish and add the capers (if using). Bake for 15 minutes. Garnish with the cilantro (if using).

Per serving: 171 calories, 5 g fat (<1 g sat fat), 22 g protein, 10 g carbohydrate, 1 g fiber, 28 mg cholesterol, 445 mg sodium

Orange Grilled Tuna

You can throw this dinner together in just 15 minutes.

SERVES 4*

1½ pounds tuna steak (sushi grade)
¼ cup frozen 100% orange juice concentrate, thawed
1 tablespoon natural honey
1 tablespoon Dijon mustard
   Pinch of salt
   Freshly ground black pepper to taste
1 teaspoon extra-virgin olive oil

1. Cut the fish into 8 equal pieces and set aside.

2. In a medium bowl, stir together the orange juice concentrate, honey, mustard, salt, and pepper. Add the fish and stir to coat.

3. Add the oil to a cast-iron grill pan and place over high heat. When the pan is very hot, add the fish and grill for 6 to 7 minutes on each side (do not overcook).

Per serving: 239 calories, 3 g fat (<1 g sat fat), 40 g protein, 11 g carbohydrate, 0 g fiber, 77 mg cholesterol, 185 mg sodium

*Serving size: 2 pieces

Lemon Salmon with Garlic Spinach

This lemony meal is fast, easy, and elegant! And let's face it, when it comes to nutrition, you can hardly do better than salmon and spinach in the same dish!

SERVES 4

4   salmon fillets (about 1½ pounds total; preferably wild Alaskan)
4   teaspoons extra-virgin olive oil
4   tablespoons lemon juice
    Salt and freshly ground black pepper (optional)
2   cloves garlic, chopped
2   bags (6 ounces each) baby spinach, rinsed

1. Preheat the broiler. Line a baking sheet with foil.

2. Place the fish on the baking sheet and drizzle each fillet evenly with 2 teaspoons of the oil and 2 tablespoons of the lemon juice. Sprinkle with salt and pepper, if desired. Broil for 10 to 12 minutes, or just until cooked through.

3. Meanwhile, heat the remaining 2 teaspoons oil in a large nonstick skillet. Add the garlic and sauté, stirring, for 20 seconds. Add the spinach several handfuls at a time. Using 2 wooden spoons, toss the spinach until it wilts. Continue until the contents of both bags fit into the skillet. Stir in the remaining 2 tablespoons lemon juice.

4. To serve, place a mound of spinach on each of 4 plates and top with a fillet.

Per serving: 357 calories, 17 g fat (3 g sat fat), 41 g protein, 10 g carbohydrate, 4 g fiber, 107 mg cholesterol, 511 mg sodium

Poached Salmon with Cucumber-Dill Sauce

This simple classic recipe is delicious hot or cold.

SERVES 4

1½ cups water

¾ cup vermouth

Juice of 1 lemon

2 tablespoons fresh dill or 2 teaspoons dry

¾ teaspoon salt

4 salmon fillets (about 1½ pounds; preferably wild Alaskan)

1½ cups fat-free plain yogurt

2 cucumbers, peeled, thinly sliced, and seeded

1 red onion, finely chopped

⅓ cup packed coarsely chopped fresh dill

2 teaspoons rice wine vinegar or apple cider vinegar

¼ teaspoon sugar

Freshly ground black pepper to taste

1. Combine the water, vermouth, lemon juice, dried dill, and ½ teaspoon of the salt in a pan large enough to hold the salmon. Bring to a gentle simmer and add the salmon. Cook for 5 to 7 minutes, or until cooked through. Transfer to a plate and discard extra liquid.

2. Meanwhile, in a medium bowl, stir together the yogurt, cucumbers, onion, fresh dill, vinegar, sugar, pepper, and the remaining salt. Serve over the poached salmon.

Per serving: 409 calories, 13 g fat (2 g sat fat), 43 g protein, 19 g carbohydrate, 1 g fiber, 109 mg cholesterol, 583 mg sodium

Poppy Seed–Crusted Salmon

Both simple and simply delicious, this quick dish cooks even faster if you replace the quinoa on the meal plan with bulgur wheat and any frozen veggie of your choice.

SERVES 4

12 Kashi TLC Original 7-Grain Crackers
4 salmon fillets (about 1½ pounds; preferably wild Alaskan)
¼ teaspoon salt
2 egg whites
2 tablespoons poppy seeds
   Freshly ground black pepper to taste
2 tablespoons extra-virgin olive oil

1. Grind the crackers in a coffee grinder or small food processor. Rinse the fish and pat dry. Salt lightly (use no more than ⅛ teaspoon of the salt).

2. In a wide, shallow dish, whisk the egg whites with a fork. On a flat plate, combine the cracker crumbs, poppy seeds, pepper, and the remaining salt.

3. One at time, dip the fillets first in the egg whites and then in the crumbs, coating both sides well.

4. Heat the oil in a large nonstick skillet. Add the fish and sear over medium-high heat for 2 to 3 minutes on each side, or until browned.

Per serving: 393 calories, 22 g fat (3 g sat fat), 42 g protein, 6 g carbohydrate, 1 g fiber, 107 mg cholesterol, 298 mg sodium

Shrimp Pasta Primavera with Basil Pesto

This tastes fantastic served cold on a summer day!

SERVES 4

- 40 frozen medium easy-peel shrimp
- 2 cups packed fresh basil leaves
- 2 tablespoons grated Parmesan or pecorino cheese
- 3 tablespoons pine nuts
- 2 cloves garlic
- $\frac{1}{4}$ teaspoon salt
- $\frac{1}{3}$ cup + 1 tablespoon extra-virgin olive oil
- 10 ounces Hodgson Mill Organic Whole Wheat Spirals with Milled Flaxseed
- 1 bag (16 ounces) frozen chopped vegetables of your choice

1. Quickly thaw the shrimp by rinsing in cold water. Peel, pat dry, and set aside.

2. In a food processor, mince the basil, cheese, pine nuts, garlic, and salt. Scrape down the sides of the bowl and drizzle in $\frac{1}{3}$ cup of the oil with the motor running. Set aside.

3. Cook the pasta according to package directions. Drain in a colander, rinse with cold water, and transfer to a large bowl.

4. Meanwhile, lightly coat a cast-iron grill pan with olive oil spray and place over high heat. When the pan is very hot, add the shrimp and grill for 2 to 3 minutes on each side (do not overcook). Add to the bowl with the pasta.

5. Add the remaining 1 tablespoon oil to the pan and sauté the frozen vegetables for a few minutes.

6. Add the vegetables and pesto to the pasta and shrimp and stir to blend.

Per serving: 606 calories, 30 g fat (4 g sat fat), 29 g protein, 59 g carbohydrate, 12 g fiber, 93 mg cholesterol, 441 mg sodium

Pineapple Shrimp

You can throw this great dish together quickly. The only time-consuming step is peeling the shrimp. If you prefer and need to cut time, use tuna steak or chicken breast cut into chunks instead.

SERVES 4

40   frozen medium shrimp

¼   cup frozen 100% pineapple juice concentrate, thawed

1   tablespoon natural honey

1   tablespoon Dijon mustard

Pinch of salt

Freshly ground black pepper to taste

2   teaspoons extra-virgin olive oil

1   cup fresh or canned unsweetened pineapple, diced

1. Quickly thaw the shrimp by rinsing in cold water. Peel, pat dry, and set aside.

2. In a medium bowl, stir together the juice concentrate, honey, mustard, salt, and pepper. Add the shrimp and stir to coat.

3. Drizzle the oil in a cast-iron grill pan and place over high heat. When the pan is very hot, add the shrimp one by one and grill for 2 to 3 minutes on each side (do not overcook). Serve with the pineapple.

Per serving: 152 calories, 4 g fat (<1 g sat fat), 12 g protein, 18 g carbohydrate, 1 g fiber, 91 mg cholesterol, 284 mg sodium

Tossed Garden Salad

Keep these ingredients on hand so you won't hesitate to throw this great salad together with dinner in a flash!

SERVES 4

SALAD

Unlimited mixed greens, baby spinach, or favorite lettuce (not iceberg)

As many raw vegetables as you can pile in a big salad bowl, such as tomatoes, cucumbers, onions, bell peppers, alfalfa sprouts, and so on. (For ease and convenience, use packaged prewashed shredded carrots, shredded cabbage-carrot coleslaw, or shredded broccoli-cabbage coleslaw.)

DRESSING

1 tablespoon extra-virgin olive oil

3 tablespoons vinegar

Pinch of salt

Freshly ground black pepper to taste

OR

5 tablespoons (5 capfuls) Newman's Own Light Italian Dressing

Build your salad any way you like!

Per serving (on average): 96 calories, 4 g fat (<1 g sat fat), 4 g protein, 13 g carbohydrate, 5 g fiber, 0 mg cholesterol, 116 mg sodium

Cucumber, Tomato, Olive, and Red Onion Salad

This classic Mediterranean salad is delicious and reminds us of blue skies and sun.

SERVES 4

2 cucumbers, sliced

1 red onion, thinly sliced

2 tomatoes, chopped

$\frac{1}{2}$ cup kalamata olives

3 tablespoons red wine vinegar

1 tablespoon extra-virgin olive oil

Pinch of salt

Freshly ground black pepper to taste

In a medium bowl, combine the cucumbers, onion, tomatoes, olives, vinegar, oil, salt, and pepper. Toss to mix.

Per serving: 128 calories, 8 g fat (1 g sat fat), 3 g protein, 12 g carbohydrate, 3 g fiber, 0 mg cholesterol, 305 mg sodium

Lentil and Bean Salad with Cilantro

This easy recipe is nutritious and very satisfying.

SERVES 4

1½ cups cooked lentils (page 229)

1 cup canned cannellini beans, rinsed and drained

1 medium tomato, chopped

1 scallion, chopped

Chopped fresh cilantro to taste

1 teaspoon + 1 tablespoon extra-virgin olive oil

2 teaspoons + 3 tablespoons balsamic vinegar

Mixed greens

Pinch of salt

Freshly ground black pepper to taste

In a large bowl, combine the lentils, beans, tomato, scallion, cilantro, 1 teaspoon of the oil, and 2 teaspoons of the vinegar. Serve over a bed of mixed greens, drizzle with the remaining 1 tablespoon oil and 3 tablespoons vinegar, and season with the salt and pepper.

Per serving: 220 calories, 6 g fat (1 g sat fat), 11 g protein, 33g carbohydrate, 8 g fiber, 0 mg cholesterol, 112 mg sodium

Minty Tabbouleh Salad

The fresh mint infuses this salad with a taste of summer. It tastes even better the next day, when the ingredients have spent some time together.

SERVES 4

4 cups cooked bulgur wheat (page 228)
2 medium tomatoes, chopped
1 can (15 ounces) chickpeas, rinsed and drained
3 scallions, chopped
  Juice of 2 lemons
1 tablespoon extra-virgin olive oil
  Pinch of onion powder
  Pinch of garlic powder
$\frac{1}{2}$ teaspoon salt
$\frac{1}{4}$ cup fresh mint, rinsed, patted dry, and chopped
2–3 cups mixed greens

In a large bowl, combine the bulgur, tomatoes, chickpeas, scallions, lemon juice, olive oil, onion powder, garlic powder, salt, and mint. Refrigerate until ready to serve over the greens.

Per serving: 275 calories, 6 g fat (<1 g sat fat), 11 g protein, 49 g carbohydrate, 13 g fiber, 0 mg cholesterol, 463 mg sodium

Pasta Fagioli with Spinach Marinara Sauce

This Italian classic features the nutritional goodness of spinach. If you orchestrate this well, you can make this dish within 15 minutes.

SERVES 4

1 tablespoon extra-virgin olive oil

4 cloves garlic, chopped

2 bags (6 ounces each) baby spinach

1 can (28 ounces) crushed tomatoes (no added oil or sugar)

1 can (15 ounces) cannellini beans, rinsed and drained

$1/2$ cup kalamata olives

1 bay leaf

1 teaspoon dried thyme

$1/4$ teaspoon salt

Freshly ground black pepper to taste

12 ounces Hodgson Mill Organic Whole Wheat Penne with Milled Flaxseed

1. Heat the oil in a large skillet. Add the garlic and sauté for a few seconds. Add the spinach one bag at a time and cook for 4 to 5 minutes, or until wilted.

2. Add the tomatoes, beans, olives, bay leaf, thyme, salt, and pepper and simmer for 8 to 10 minutes.

3. Meanwhile, cook the pasta according to package directions. Drain in a colander and transfer to a bowl. Remove the bay leaf from the sauce and serve over the pasta.

Per serving: 568 calories, 12 g fat (1 g sat fat), 24 g protein, 102 g carbohydrate, 21 g fiber, 0 mg cholesterol, 971 mg sodium

Pasta with Marinara Sauce

What could be simpler than this classic tomato dinner?

SERVES 4

1   tablespoon extra-virgin olive oil

4   cloves garlic, chopped

1   can (28 ounces) crushed tomatoes (no added oil or sugar)

1   teaspoon dried thyme or oregano

1   bay leaf

¼   teaspoon salt

    Freshly ground black pepper to taste

12   ounces Hodgson Mill Whole Wheat Spaghetti

2   tablespoons grated Parmesan cheese

1. Heat the oil in a deep skillet. Add the garlic and sauté for a few seconds.

2. Add the tomatoes, thyme, bay leaf, salt, and pepper and simmer for 8 to 10 minutes.

3. Meanwhile, cook the pasta according to package directions. Drain in a colander and transfer to a bowl. Remove the bay leaf from the sauce and serve over the pasta, sprinkled with the cheese.

Per serving: 397 calories, 6 g fat (1 g sat fat), 18 g protein, 76 g carbohydrate, 13 g fiber, 2 mg cholesterol, 469 mg sodium

Apple–Butternut Squash Soup

*This soup is very creamy even though it's very low in fat. The sweet flavor of apple
intensifies if you make it in advance and refrigerate it before pureeing.*

SERVES 4

    2 teaspoons extra-virgin olive oil
    1 large yellow onion, finely chopped
    2 teaspoons mild curry powder
 $^3/_4$ teaspoon salt
 $1^1/_4$ pounds butternut squash*, chopped
    2 medium apples, peeled, cored, and cut into large chunks
    3 cups fat-free chicken broth
 $^3/_4$ cup apple cider
 $1^1/_2$ cups fat-free buttermilk

1. Heat the oil in a soup pot over medium heat. Reduce the heat to low, add
   the onion and curry, and sauté for 8 to 10 minutes, or until tender.

2. When the onion is tender, add the salt, squash, apples, and broth and bring
   to a boil. Reduce the heat, add the apple cider, and simmer for about 20
   minutes, until the squash and apples are very tender. Remove from the
   heat and let stand for a few minutes.

3. Pour the soup in batches into a blender or food processor and puree until
   smooth. Return to the pot, add the buttermilk, and simmer briefly to heat
   through.

Per serving: 225 calories, 3 g fat (< 1 g sat fat), 10 g protein, 42 g carbohydrate, 8 g fiber,
0 mg cholesterol, 659 mg sodium

*Look for it peeled and precut, frozen, or bagged fresh in the produce section.

Satisfaction at the Flavor Point

THE FLAVOR FACTS

Name: Jim Butler

Age: 39

Hometown: Derby, Connecticut

Family status: Married with two children, ages 7 and 8

Occupation: Security, telecom, safety, and facilities supervisor; Derby fire chief

Starting weight: 325

Pounds lost: 31 in 12 weeks

Health stats: Blood pressure dropped 19 points; blood sugar dropped 15 points; lost 4 inches from waist; over 5 percent decline in body fat

"I was diagnosed with Guillain-Barré syndrome, paralyzed from the waist down, and hospitalized for a week in August 2004. After I was discharged, things went downhill fast. My food consumption went way up, my energy went down, and I gained 68 pounds. I felt like a slug—fat, with no energy. I was eating 7,000-plus calories, including two or three servings of red meat per day. I was the perfect example of how not to eat. I would get out of a meeting at 10:00 p.m. and stop at McDonald's for two or three double cheeseburgers . . . for a snack. I had to do something!

"Prior to starting this program, I, as well as my whole family, would eat in order to not feel hungry. I was living to eat rather than eating to live.

"I work full-time and am the fire chief here in Derby, so I'm pretty busy. I wasn't sure I'd have the time to follow a meal plan, but I made the commitment to do it. My health was at stake.

"To keep myself going in the beginning, I decided not to weigh myself for the first 2 weeks. When I had to move down a belt hole, I knew it was time to step on the scale. In the first 2 weeks, I lost 21 pounds! I was very pleased at that point, and I have been ever since.

"I like the flavor themes on Dr. Katz's program, particularly the pineapple and nuts. And the bulgur wheat was by far my best new find. I eat it with everything. For a snack (or even a late-night fix if I need it), the bulgur mixed with yogurt is great.

"I wish I had changed my eating habits years ago. I have not had red meat in 12 weeks, and I don't miss it at all. When I go to parties or gatherings, I have a salad. My eating habits have changed 100 percent. Now I eat real food.

"Many people have commented on my weight loss, saying, 'You look great!' and asking me how much I've lost. Everyone asks me about the diet I'm on, and I always explain it the same way: It is a serious lifestyle change, and you need to approach it as such. You need to stay focused; if you do, and you combine a little exercise with it, the results are astounding.

"Today, I feel great. I have lots more energy, and I only expect to get more as the pounds continue to come off. I don't consider this a diet as much as I do a way to eat well.

"Although I have to admit I was a little skeptical at first, I'm so happy I've stuck with Dr. Katz's program. I was a walking time bomb, and if I had gone on one of those fad diets, I think I would have given up a long time ago. Those are diets; this is a lifestyle change." ■

Portobello Mushrooms with Walnut Stuffing

This dish requires a little more preparation than most other Flavor Point recipes. You can prepare the mushrooms in advance and refrigerate them so you can just pop them in the oven when you're ready.

SERVES 4*

8	medium or 4 large portobello mushroom caps
15	Kashi TLC Original 7-Grain Crackers
2	teaspoons extra-virgin olive oil
1	small yellow onion, chopped
2	cloves garlic, chopped
1	stalk celery, chopped
6	baby carrots, chopped
$\frac{1}{3}$	cup chopped walnuts
$\frac{3}{4}$	cup bulgur wheat (dry)
2	cups fat-free chicken broth
1	teaspoon dried thyme
	Pinch of salt
	Freshly ground black pepper to taste
$\frac{1}{4}$	cup grated Parmesan or Asiago cheese
1	teaspoon ground paprika

1. Preheat the oven to 375°F. Coat a baking dish with olive oil spray.

2. Rinse the mushrooms, pat dry, and trim the stems (there's no need to hollow out the caps). Set aside.

3. Grind the crackers in a coffee grinder or small food processor. Set aside.

4. Heat the oil in a nonstick skillet over medium heat. Add the onion, garlic, celery, and carrots and sauté for 2 to 3 minutes.

5. Add the bulgur and cook, stirring, for a few seconds. Add the broth and cook until the bulgur is tender and all the liquid is absorbed. Remove from the heat and stir in the thyme, cracker crumbs, walnuts, salt, and pepper.

6. Place the mushrooms in the baking dish and use an ice cream scoop to fill them with the stuffing mixture, packing it down slightly (they'll be over-stuffed, but that's okay!).

7. Sprinkle the tops with the cheese and paprika and coat lightly with olive oil spray. Bake for 15 to 20 minutes.

Per serving: 341 calories, 13 g fat (2 g sat fat), 15 g protein, 43 g carbohydrate, 8 g fiber, 6 mg cholesterol, 381 mg sodium

*Serving size: 2 medium mushrooms or 1 large

Mint, Sweet Pea, and Spinach Soup

Catherine adapted this recipe from an old-time favorite from The Silver Palate Cook-book. *She was skeptical when she first discovered it years ago but was won over by the delicious blend of flavors, so here it is with a few healthy changes that preserve its creaminess. It's quick and easy to put together, as long as you have a blender!*

SERVES 4

2   tablespoons extra-virgin olive oil

2   cups finely chopped yellow onion

2   bags (10 ounces each) frozen chopped spinach, thawed

2   bags (10 ounces each) frozen peas, thawed

4   cups fat-free chicken broth

2   cups packed fresh mint

3/4   teaspoon salt

    Freshly ground black pepper to taste

1 3/4   cups fat-free buttermilk

1. Heat the oil in a soup pot. Add the onions and sauté for about 5 minutes, or until soft.

2. Add the spinach, peas, and broth and bring to a boil. Reduce the heat and simmer for 10 to 12 minutes. Add the mint, salt, and pepper, remove from the heat, and let stand for a few minutes.

3. Pour the soup in batches into a food processor or blender and process until smooth. Return to the pan, add the buttermilk, and simmer briefly, stirring, to heat through.

Per serving: 315 calories, 8 g fat (1 g sat fat), 23 g protein, 40 g carbohydrate, 13 g fiber, 0 mg cholesterol, 972 mg sodium

Pumpkin Soup

This soup takes 8 minutes to make from opening the cans to putting it on the table.
It's so creamy and satisfying you could swear it was made with pure cream!
It's perfect on a fall evening.

SERVES 4

2 teaspoons extra-virgin olive oil

1 teaspoon minced fresh ginger or garlic

4 cans (15 ounces each) pumpkin (no added salt or sugar)

3 cups fat-free vegetable or chicken broth

2 cups fat-free buttermilk

$^1/_2$ teaspoon salt

$^1/_4$ cup light unsweetened coconut milk

1. Heat the oil in a soup pot over medium heat. Add the ginger or garlic and sauté for 1 minute.

2. Add the pumpkin, broth, buttermilk, and salt and stir. Simmer for 5 to 7 minutes, or until hot.

3. To serve, ladle the soup into 4 bowls and drizzle a swirl of coconut milk on top of each.

Per serving: 242 calories, 4 g fat (2 g sat fat), 14 g protein, 41 g carbohydrate, 12 g fiber, 0 mg cholesterol, 553 mg sodium

Dill Potatoes

Fresh dill is the perfect complement to steamed potatoes. Used frequently in potato salads, dill lets you avoid the calories and saturated fat that come with potato's other customary partners—butter and sour cream!

SERVES 4

3 medium red potatoes, cut into chunks
2 teaspoons extra-virgin olive oil
1 tablespoon fresh dill
   Pinch of salt

1. Steam the potatoes until tender.

2. In a small bowl, combine the oil, dill, and salt.

3. Place the potatoes in a serving bowl and drizzle with the oil.

Per serving: 137 calories, 3g fat (0 g sat fat), 3 g protein, 26 g carbohydrate, 2 g fiber, 0 mg cholesterol, 156 mg sodium

Sautéed Spaghetti Squash

This squash can also be served as is right out of the microwave,
drizzled with olive oil.

SERVES 4

1   medium spaghetti squash
2   teaspoons extra-virgin olive oil
    Pinch of salt
    Freshly ground black pepper to taste

1. Pierce the rind of the squash with a fork and microwave on high for 10 to 12 minutes (or 5 to 6 minutes per pound) until the skin feels soft. Cut in half and remove the seeds. Twist out the strands with a fork.

2. Heat the oil in a nonstick skillet. Add the squash and sauté until heated through. Season with the salt and pepper.

Per serving: 84 calories, 3 g fat (<1 g sat fat), 2 g protein, 15 g carbohydrate, 3 g fiber, 0 mg cholesterol, 115 mg sodium

Roasted Asparagus with Pecans and Sun-Dried Tomatoes

Along with rich, enticing flavor, pecans add healthful unsaturated oils and vitamin E to this dish.

SERVES 4

1 pound asparagus (the thin kind in a bunch)
1 tablespoon chopped pecans
3 tablespoons oil-packed julienned sun-dried tomatoes, drained
1 teaspoon extra-virgin olive oil
$1/4$ teaspoon salt

1. Preheat the oven to 375°F. Cut $1/2$ inch off the ends of the asparagus. Rinse the spears and pat dry.

2. In a small baking dish, drizzle the asparagus, pecans, and tomatoes with the oil and sprinkle with the salt. Stir to mix.

3. Bake for 8 to 10 minutes, or until the asparagus is crisp-tender.

Per serving: 65 calories, 3 g fat (0 g sat fat), 3 g protein, 6 g carbohydrate, 3 g fiber, 0 mg cholesterol, 159 mg sodium

Whole Wheat Garlic Bread

Yes, you can even eat garlic bread on the Flavor Point Diet, as long as you make it with whole grain bread.

SERVES 4

1   loaf (16 ounces) whole wheat Italian bread
2   teaspoons extra-virgin olive oil
1   clove garlic, crushed

Cut the bread in half lengthwise, then drizzle one half with the olive oil and top with the garlic (freeze the other half for another day). Bake at 375°F until browned, then cut into 4 slices.

Per serving: 122 calories, 3 g fat (0 g sat fat), 3 g protein, 24 g carbohydrate, 8 g fiber, 0 mg cholesterol, 134 mg sodium

COOKED WHOLE GRAINS AND LENTILS

Brown Rice

More flavorful than white rice, brown rice is also much more nutritious; in particular, it's an excellent source of fiber.

MAKES ABOUT 4 CUPS

5 cups water (scant)

1¹/₂ cups brown rice

Bring the water to a boil in a large saucepan. Add the rice and cook for about 15 minutes, or until tender.

Per serving: 258 calories, 2 g fat (0 g sat fat), 5 g protein, 54 g carbohydrate, 2 g fiber, 0 mg cholesterol, 9 mg sodium

Bulgur Wheat

Bulgur wheat has no fat and is relatively low in calories and high in fiber and protein. It takes all of 5 minutes to make (much less time than pasta or rice), never clumps, and is always "forgiving" if you boil it in a little too much water. On top of that, kids love it! The rule of thumb is simple: Use almost twice as much water (but not quite: It's a 1:1³/₄ ratio) as dry bulgur.

MAKES ABOUT 4 CUPS

3 cups water (scant)

1¹/₂ cups bulgur wheat

Bring the water to a boil in a medium saucepan. Add the bulgur and cook for 5 minutes. Let cool, then refrigerate in an airtight container for 1 week.

Per serving: 180 calories, <1 g fat (0 g sat fat), 6 g protein, 40 g carbohydrate, 10 g fiber, 0 mg cholesterol, 14 mg sodium

Lentils

Lentils are so good for everyone's health that having them already cooked in the fridge may encourage the rest of your family to eat them more often!

MAKES 4 CUPS

1½ cups dry lentils
5 cups water

1. Rinse and drain the lentils.

2. Bring the water to a boil in a large saucepan. Add the lentils and cook for 10 to 15 minutes, or until tender but not mushy. Drain in a colander and rinse with cold water. Refrigerate in an airtight container for 1 week.

Per serving: 243 calories, 0 g fat (0 g sat fat), 20 g protein, 41 g carbohydrate, 22 g fiber, 0 mg cholesterol, 7 mg sodium

Quinoa

This nutritious, delicious grain keeps well in the fridge, precooked, and won't clump even when reheated in the microwave. It's great as a side dish alone or can be mixed with bulgur wheat. It takes roughly 10 minutes longer to cook than bulgur.

MAKES ABOUT 3 CUPS

4½ cups water
1½ cups quinoa

Bring the water to a boil in a large saucepan. Add the quinoa and cook for 12 to 15 minutes, or until tender. Drain if necessary. Let cool, then refrigerate in an airtight container for 1 week.

Per serving: 238 calories, 4 g fat (0 g sat fat), 8 g protein, 44 g carbohydrate, 4 g fiber, 0 mg cholesterol, 13 mg sodium

DESSERTS

Baked Bananas
with Rum-Pecan Topping

This quick and easy version of bananas Foster features the buttery taste of pecans.

SERVES 4*

$\frac{1}{4}$ cup pecans

1 tablespoon rum

1 tablespoon water

1 tablespoon dark brown sugar

2 ripe bananas, halved lengthwise[†]

1. Preheat a toaster oven to 350°F. Coarsely grind the pecans in a small food processor.

2. In a small bowl, combine the rum, water, brown sugar, and pecans. Drizzle over each banana half.

3. Bake for 5 to 7 minutes, then broil for 1 minute, or until the top is sizzling.

Per serving: 129 calories, 6 g fat (<1 g sat fat), 1 g protein, 18 g carbohydrate, 2 g fiber, 0 mg cholesterol, 2 mg sodium

*Serving size: $\frac{1}{2}$ banana

[†]Keep the skin on so you can serve it right from its "shell."

Baked Cinnamon Apples

This dessert is as heartwarming as it is delicious.

SERVES 4

2 apples, halved and cored

2 tablespoons apple cider

2 teaspoons dark brown sugar

Pinch of ground cinnamon

1. Preheat a toaster oven to 350°F. Line the toaster oven tray with foil and place the apples on the tray, core side up.

2. In a cup, combine the cider, brown sugar, and cinnamon. Drizzle over the apples.

3. Bake for 10 to 12 minutes, then broil for 1 minute, or until the top is sizzling.

Per serving: 53 calories, 0 g fat (0 g sat fat), 0 g protein, 14 g carbohydrate, 2 g fiber, 0 mg cholesterol, 2 mg sodium

VARIATIONS

Baked Cinnamon-Almond Apples: Add $\frac{1}{4}$ cup chopped almonds in step 2.

Per serving: 88 calories, 3 g fat (0 g sat fat), 1 g protein, 15 g carbohydrate, 3 g fiber, 0 mg cholesterol, 2 mg sodium

Baked Cinnamon-Walnut Apples: Add $\frac{1}{4}$ cup chopped walnuts in step 2.

Per serving: 86 calories, 4 g fat (0 g sat fat), 1 g protein, 14 g carbohydrate, 2 g fiber, 0 mg cholesterol, 2 mg sodium

Chocolate Brownies

These moist little brownies taste as rich and chewy as they sound, yet they contain no added butter or oil! Tofu is the magic ingredient, but your family will never know it's there. Be sure to cut them into exactly 24 squares and have only 1 per person. (Freeze the rest for another specialty indulgence day!)

MAKES 24 BROWNIES (2" SQUARES)

- $\frac{1}{3}$ cup almonds
- $\frac{1}{2}$ cup fat-free milk
- 4 ounces Ghirardelli bittersweet chocolate
- $\frac{3}{4}$ cup soft silken tofu (about $\frac{1}{3}$ of a 14-ounce package), extra water discarded
- 3 eggs
- $\frac{1}{2}$ cup nonfat dry milk
- 2 tablespoons unsweetened cocoa
- $\frac{1}{3}$ cup packed dark brown sugar
- $\frac{1}{4}$ cup soft wheat pastry flour*
- $\frac{1}{2}$ teaspoon baking powder
- $\frac{2}{3}$ cup Ghirardelli Double Chocolate Chips
- 1–2 teaspoons confectioners' sugar, sifted (optional)

1. Preheat the oven to 325°F. Grind the almonds in a coffee grinder or small food processor.

2. Bring the fat-free milk to a boil in a small saucepan, then remove from the heat. Break up the chocolate, add to the milk, and stir until creamy. Set aside.

3. Place the tofu, eggs, dry milk, cocoa, and brown sugar in the bowl of an electric mixer and beat until well blended.

4. Add the melted chocolate and beat until blended. Add the ground almonds, flour, and baking powder and beat until well blended. Stir in the chocolate chips.

5. Pour the batter into an ungreased 12¼" × 8¼" × 1¼" cake pan (foil pans work well) and bake for 15 to 20 minutes. When cool, sift the confectioners' sugar (if using) on top and cut into 24 squares.

Per brownie: 98 calories, 5 g fat (2 g sat fat), 3 g protein, 12 g carbohydrate, 1 g fiber, 23 mg cholesterol, 30 mg sodium

*Arrowhead Mills Organic Pastry Flour or any other brand of soft wheat (not whole wheat) flour with fiber is fine. You can also use Hodgson Mill Oat Bran Flour.

Caramelized Pineapple Rings

This simple, quick, and delicious dish provides a perfect ending to Pineapple Day.

SERVES 4

8   fresh or canned unsweetened pineapple rings

4   teaspoons brown sugar

1. Spread the pineapple in a single layer on a baking sheet and sprinkle the brown sugar evenly over the top.

2. Broil for 3 to 5 minutes, or until caramelized.

Per serving: 77 calories, 0 g fat (0 g sat fat), 0 g protein, 20 g carbohydrate, 1 g fiber, 0 mg cholesterol, 12 mg sodium

Peach Flat Cake

This cake is similar to the luscious, buttery galettes from Brittany in the north of France, except, of course, it has no butter! Its dense flat batter topped with fresh peaches rises slightly as it bakes to embrace the fruit, so it's not only delicious, it's also beautiful. Surprisingly, it's quick and simple to make. Freeze any leftovers and save for another Peach Day.

SERVES 6*

$\frac{1}{2}$	teaspoon + $\frac{1}{4}$ cup Smart Balance spread
$\frac{1}{4}$	cup nonfat dry milk
$\frac{1}{4}$	cup granulated sugar
1	tablespoon sliced almonds
2	eggs
$\frac{1}{4}$	cup soft wheat pastry flour†
$\frac{1}{4}$	teaspoon baking powder
2	medium ripe peaches, peeled and thinly sliced, or 1 can (8 ounces) juice-packed sliced peaches, drained

1. Preheat the oven to 350°F. Grease the bottom of a round cake pan with $\frac{1}{2}$ teaspoon of the spread.

2. Place the dry milk, sugar, almonds, and the remaining $\frac{1}{4}$ cup spread in the bowl of an electric mixer and beat on medium speed until creamy. Add the eggs and beat for a few minutes, or until the batter is "airy." Add the flour and baking powder and mix again until well blended.

3. Pour batter into the pan and lay the peaches in a circle on top. Bake for 20 minutes, or until golden.

Per serving: 151 calories, 9 g fat (2 g sat fat), 4 g protein, 16 g carbohydrate, 1 g fiber, 60 mg cholesterol, 118 mg sodium

*Serving size: 1 slice

†Arrowhead Mills Organic Pastry Flour or any other brand of soft wheat (not whole wheat) flour with fiber is fine. You can also use Hodgson Mill Oat Bran Flour.

Satisfaction at the Flavor Point

THE FLAVOR FACTS

Name: Jonathan Link

Age: 33

Hometown: Derby, Connecticut

Family status: Single

Occupation: Software engineer

Starting weight: 178

Pounds lost: 15 in 12 weeks

Health stats: Cholesterol dropped 72 points; waist measurement shrank $4^{1}/_{2}$ inches; 7 percent decline in body fat

"Before starting Dr. Katz's program, I could not hold myself to a reasonable portion size. I would empty a whole box of cereal into a container that looked like a trough, and that was my breakfast. Throughout my life, I had always been pretty thin—fluctuating between 155 and 160. Once I hit my thirties, however, I started working first shift instead of third and started eating more and exercising less. It caught up with me.

"When I first saw how much cereal I really should be eating, I was like, 'Get out of here—that's it?' I thought I'd be hungry on the program all the time. I was wrong. In fact, I never felt hungry. After week 2, I couldn't eat everything. I only made three of the desserts throughout the entire program—two fruit salads and a peach flatbread (which was delicious!)—because I was too full to eat them.

"I'm a pretty eclectic eater (I eat everything except internal organs), so I had tried most of the foods on the program before. The food was excellent. I remember a grilled pumpkin and chocolate panini I had for lunch one day. It was to die for. I thought, 'There is no possible way this is good for me—it's too delicious and decadent.'

"I also loved the way Catherine Katz incorporated so many different textures into the dishes, like nuts and cranberries sprinkled on a salad. It goes along with my philosophy that eating should really be a whole experience; food can't just taste good—it has to look good and feel good in your mouth, too. Otherwise everything would just be like applesauce.

"Although all the recipes were really good, I think I enjoyed the chicken ones the best. I was surprised at some of the ingredients in the dishes. When I looked over the meal plan, I thought there was no way these things would taste good together. Again, I was wrong. The combinations were consistently delicious.

"I also learned how to make a bunch of simple sauces. When I used to cook for myself, I'd skip the sauce because I thought it would take forever. Now that I've learned how to and gotten in the habit of doing it, I know all I have to do is take whatever I cooked with and work with it for a few more seconds to make a great sauce—one that tastes as delicious as something I would eat at a restaurant.

"I also learned many great new tricks that I will definitely use for the rest of my life. For instance, when it came to salad dressings, I was always a Wish-Bone kind of guy. When I saw that I had to squeeze an orange on my chicken salad, I thought, 'This isn't going to be good,' but it tasted great! Now, I figure there's no sense in buying salad dressings if I can make my own. I used to be a mayonnaise freak. When I tried the fat-free yogurt in chicken salad instead of mayonnaise, it was awesome. I loved it. I'll probably never eat mayo again because the yogurt is so much healthier and it tastes just as good.

"When I eat out, I have to admit, I've become one of those people I used to hate—I order the plain chicken and the salad with the dressing on the side—because you know what? I'm paying for it, and I should be able to have it the way I want it. I used to be able to eat a whole fast-food value meal and still be hungry for something else, and now I eat one veggie burger and I can't even eat the fries.

"I'm definitely going to stay on Dr. Katz's program, and I will advertise it like it's going out of style—I'm a walking advertisement for it! If you stick with it, you can't fail. There is no way for you to follow these recipes and not lose weight and feel great about yourself in the process. It's a can't-fail plan."

Piña Colada Frozen Dessert

This fun, easy tropical dessert will make you feel as if you are relaxing on a sunny island.

SERVES 4

$^1/_2$ cup light unsweetened coconut milk

2 cups crushed pineapple in its own juice (preferably fresh)

2 tablespoons dark rum

1 cup crushed ice

Place the coconut milk, pineapple, rum, and ice in a blender and process until smooth. Pour into 4 individual bowls or glasses and place in the freezer for at least 15 minutes before serving.

Per serving: 110 calories, 2 g fat (1 g sat fat), <1 g protein, 21 g carbohydrate, 1 g fiber, 0 mg cholesterol, 9 mg sodium

Peanut Katz Flax Crisps

These no-bake cookies are a healthy and nutritious alternative to conventional Rice Krispies treats, which typically contain no fiber, lots of saturated and hydrogenated fat, and marshmallow sugar goo! Instead, these little squares are filled with the healthy omega-3 fatty acids found in flaxseed and, with the peanut butter and organic crispy brown rice cereal, are a great source of dietary fiber. They freeze well, so keep them handy, and remember to stick to 1 square per person.

MAKES 30 SQUARES

1 cup natural honey

1 cup natural peanut butter*

1 cup dark flaxseed[†]

5–5$^1/_2$ cups Erewhon Crispy Brown Rice Cereal

$^1/_3$ cup Ghirardelli semisweet chocolate chips

1. Heat the honey in a pan over low heat for 2 to 3 minutes, or until warm and slightly liquefied. Remove from the heat and stir in the peanut butter until melted and smooth.

2. Finely grind the flaxseed ¹/₂ cup at a time in a coffee grinder. Place in a large bowl with 4 cups of the cereal and mix gently with clean hands.

3. Add the warm peanut butter–honey mixture and stir well with a spoon. Add the remaining 1¹/₂ cups cereal, ¹/₂ cup at a time (if it gets too hard to stir at the end, you may leave out ¹/₂ cup). Stir in the chocolate chips while still warm.

4. Pour into an ungreased 12¹/₄" × 8¹/₄" × 1¹/₄" cake pan (foil pans work well) and press down to flatten with slightly damp, clean hands until nicely compact and flat throughout. Refrigerate for 15 minutes and cut into 30 squares.

Per serving: 146 calories, 7 g fat (1 g sat fat), 3 g protein, 19 g carbohydrate, 2 g fiber, 0 mg cholesterol, 61 mg sodium

*Some of the natural oils in unprocessed peanut butter accumulate on top before its first use. Discard the oil when opening a new jar to lower the fat content.

†To fully benefit from the healthy nutritional value of the omega-3's in flaxseed, it's best to grind it fresh, but it's fine to use ground flax meal.

Raisin-Granola Parfait

Refrigerate this dessert for at least 30 minutes after assembling and before serving, as each layer becomes infused with the other. Be sure to follow the amounts specified in the recipe and not get carried away with the raisins and the granola!

SERVES 4

1 cup low-fat granola
4 tablespoons raisins or currants
1 cup fat-free vanilla yogurt
1 cup fat-free plain yogurt

1. Grind the granola in a coffee grinder, then grind the raisins or currants.

2. In a small bowl, stir together the vanilla and plain yogurt until creamy.

3. Line up 4 tall, thin glasses. Spoon 1 tablespoon of the yogurt into each glass, then add a sprinkle of granola and a sprinkle of raisins. Continue alternating layers, ending with the granola. Use a total of $1/2$ cup of yogurt for each glass. Refrigerate for at least 30 minutes before serving (you can also freeze it if you prefer).

Per serving: 187 calories, 1 g fat (0 g sat fat), 8 g protein, 39 g carbohydrate, 2 g fiber, 3 mg cholesterol, 131 mg sodium

Strawberries Dipped in Dark Chocolate

Although it tastes decadently delicious, this is in fact a very nutritious treat!

SERVES 1

- 1 ounce bittersweet chocolate
- 4 large strawberries
- 4 teaspoons fat-free milk

1. Break up the chocolate. Rinse and dry the strawberries.

2. In a small microwaveable bowl, microwave the chocolate and milk on medium-high for 25 seconds, or until melted. Stir until creamy and let cool for a few minutes before dipping the strawberries.

Per serving: 198 calories, 10 g fat (6 g sat fat), 3 g protein, 25 g carbohydrate, 5 g fiber, 1 mg cholesterol, 13 mg sodium

Warm Apple Crisp

A classic quick and simple dessert!

SERVES 4

$\frac{1}{2}$ cup low-fat nutty granola

2 teaspoons Smart Balance spread

3 apples, rinsed, cored, and thickly sliced

$\frac{1}{3}$ cup apple cider

1 tablespoon chopped almonds

1 tablespoon brown sugar

Pinch of cinnamon

1. Preheat the oven to 350°F.

2. Finely grind the granola in a coffee grinder or small food processor.

3. Spread the Smart Balance in the bottom of a shallow baking dish and arrange the apples in a single layer.

4. Pour the cider over the apples and sprinkle with the granola, almonds, brown sugar, and cinnamon.

5. Bake for 15 to 20 minutes, or until the apples are tender.

Per serving: 163 calories, 4 g fat (<1 g sat fat), 2 g protein, 33 g carbohydrate, 4 g fiber, 0 mg cholesterol, 52 mg sodium

Mint Chocolate Chip Shake

So minty, delicious, and satisfying, you'll forget you're on a diet.

SERVES 4

1½ cups low-fat vanilla frozen yogurt
1 cup fat-free milk
1 tablespoon Ghirardelli semisweet chocolate chips
Drop of peppermint extract

In a blender, process the yogurt, milk, chocolate chips, and peppermint until smooth.

Per serving: 118 calories, 1 g fat (<1 g sat fat), 6 g protein, 21 g carbohydrate, 0 g fiber, 0 mg cholesterol, 84 mg sodium

Cranberry-Vanilla Soft Ice Cream

Deliciously tart, this dessert provides a perfect ending to Cranberry Day.

SERVES 4*

2 cups fat-free vanilla ice cream or frozen yogurt
⅓ cup fat-free milk
2 tablespoons fresh or frozen cranberries

In a blender, process the ice cream, milk, and cranberries until smooth.

Per serving: 97 calories, 0 g fat (0 g sat fat), 5 g protein, 19 g carbohydrate, 0 g fiber, 2 mg cholesterol, 64 mg sodium

*Serving size: ½ cup

Pumpkin Soft Ice Cream

If you love pumpkin pie, you'll love this tasty ice cream dessert.

SERVES 4

2   cups fat-free vanilla ice cream

2   tablespoons canned pureed pumpkin (no added salt or sugar)

¼   cup fat-free milk

Pinch of allspice

In a blender, process the ice cream, pumpkin, milk, and allspice until smooth.

Per serving: 98 calories, 0 g fat (0 g sat fat), 4 g protein, 20 g carbohydrate, 1 g fiber, 0 mg cholesterol, 74 mg sodium

6

STAYING ON POINT FOR LIFE

You've graduated from the school of flavor themes. You no longer need them as long as you adhere to the Flavor Point principles.

Learning to lower your Flavor Point is similar to learning to ride a bike. In the beginning, you needed training wheels—in the form of flavor themes—to guide your eating and balance your appetite. Now, after spending 6 weeks using the Flavor Point Meal Plan, you're ready to dispose of the training wheels as you continue to pedal toward your weight-loss goal.

How do you avoid falling? How do you permanently maintain the Flavor Point benefits without flavor themes? Without necessarily even realizing it, you have *already* learned all the principles you need to balance at the Flavor Point—permanently. Here's a quick recap of how you traveled from point A to point B.

In phase 1 of the meal plan, you followed daylong flavor themes to subdue your appetite.

During this phase, you also began eating meals and snacks that were wholesome, minimally processed, and free of unnecessary flavors. As you gained mastery over Flavor Point principles—learning to choose Flavor Point–approved foods and cook Flavor Point–worthy meals—you were able to decrease your dependence on the flavor themes. That's why, in phase 2 of the plan, you ate a greater variety of flavors over the course of each day, limiting your flavor themes to individual meals. Thus, you learned how to have variety *over time* without having too much variety *at any one time.*

That is a crucial Flavor Point principle that you must stick with for a lifetime in order to reach and maintain your goal. Over time, you can have all the variety you want. Savory foods, salty foods, sweet foods, and spicy foods are all fine; you just can't eat them all at once! Go ahead and enjoy slightly sweetened whole grain cereal for breakfast along with sweet fruit. Have a savory bean salad at lunch with flavor-neutral whole grain bread. At dinner, eat a slightly spicy, herb-encrusted fish fillet or chicken breast with a flavor-neutral salad. That's variety over time.

On the other hand, don't eat a breakfast of salted eggs with sweet jam on toast. Don't have a savory cheese or meat sandwich with salty potato chips and sweet soda at lunch. Don't snack on sweet fruit *and* salted nuts. These are all examples of too much variety at any one time.

To adhere to this principle, distribute flavors over the course of each day according to the following guidelines.

Breakfast. Combine a flavor-neutral food with either a sweet or salty food. For example, try grains with sweet fruit (see day 1 of the meal plan on page 78 for an example) or salted eggs with flavor-neutral whole grain bread *without* sweet jam (see day 18 on page 99).

Midmorning snack. Have sweet fruit with a dairy product (see day 36 on page 120) and don't have savory or salty items.

Lunch. Eat either savory and/or salty foods, but not sweet ones. For example, you can have a turkey sandwich on whole grain bread with lettuce, tomato, and mustard (see day 21 on page 102).

Midafternoon snack. Snack on items with savory and/or salty flavors, but don't have sweet items. For example, lightly salted nuts are a great snack (see day 19 on page 100).

Dinner. Use the same simple sauce or dressing on your main course as you do on your side dish (see day 4 on page 81).

Dessert. If you have dessert, keep it simple. Try a bit of plain dark chocolate or a fruit salad. Consider having a flavor for dessert that you had at dinner, such as orange sorbet following a dinner that used orange in a sauce (see day 17 on page 98).

In addition to being aware of how you combine the flavors in your meals and snacks, you must also pay attention to the individual brands and products that you eat. As you've learned, many packaged foods have too many conflicting flavors. After using the meal plan for 6 weeks, you have developed the habit of choosing wholesome, conveniently available products and brands that do not contain excess flavors. (To further guide your choices, consult the appendix for dozens of foods with the Flavor Point seal of approval.) In general, you will steer clear of foods with long ingredient lists and artificial flavors, sweet foods with significant additions of salt, and salty foods with significant additions of sugar.

REDIRECTING RECIPES TO THE FLAVOR POINT

You can apply Flavor Point strategies to your preparation of favorite family recipes, improving their nutritional value and cutting out unnecessary flavor additions while preserving their familiar taste and appearance. This process, of course, involves some trial and error. Keep in mind that while most dishes stand up very well to ingredient substitutions or are even improved by them, the occasional dish tastes palatable only when you follow the original recipe. To modify existing recipes to conform to Flavor Point guidelines, you will reduce sugar in baked goods, reduce salt in sweet foods, and lower fat and increase fiber in many of your recipes. You will also avoid using highly processed ingredients that contain artificial flavor enhancers. In the following pages, you'll find numerous substitutions—along with recipes for guidance—to help you do just that.

Satisfaction at the Flavor Point

THE FLAVOR FACTS

Name: Donna Durmazlar

Age: 38

Hometown: Milford, Connecticut

Family status: Married with two children, ages 15 and 21

Occupation: Nursing staff coordinator

Starting weight: 207

Pounds lost: 10 in 12 weeks

Health stats: Blood pressure dropped 17 points; lost ½ inch off waist

"I grew up in a household where you could never find cookies or ice cream, and we only had soda on the holidays. My mother made us finish our vegetables before we could eat any other part of our dinner. It was good for me at the time, but it really made me rebel. For the past 25 years, I've eaten whatever I wanted, and it usually wasn't vegetables.

"As a result, I gained 50 pounds with my first pregnancy (way back in 1989!), and then during the past 3 years, I gained another 20. I tried Weight Watchers in 1998 and lost about 35 pounds, but I got lazy, didn't stick with it, and gained it all back. I started to get really sick of being overweight, so I decided to try Dr. Katz's program.

"When I first began the program and Dr. Katz said, 'Don't think of this as a diet but as a way of eating,' I didn't quite get it. Now I truly understand what he meant and have adopted his philosophy.

"I have to admit, the first week was an adjustment, but after that, I was fine. My biggest temptation is chocolate, and when I got to Chocolate Day, I was beside myself—I was like, 'Oh, my God . . . you can have chocolate on this diet?' Better yet, I always feel satisfied. I haven't made many of the desserts called for on the meal plan because I'm usually too full. And my tastes have changed—I *want* more wholesome foods.

"Not only are the foods and recipes delicious, they're also healthful. I never knew there were so many foods out there that are good for you and still have so much flavor. The crackers on the program taste just like my favorite wheat crackers, but they are, of course, much healthier. I never would have thought to cook with fruit before, but it makes everything so sweet; it's pretty much a substitute for sugar. Catherine Katz definitely put a lot of thought and creativity into the program to make the recipes tasty. Overall, I have to say the Pistachio-Crusted Chicken is my favorite.

"Schedule-wise, I'm pretty busy, so I follow the flavor-friendly options for breakfast and lunch. For breakfast, I have cereal or fruit, and for lunch, I have a salad with chicken or tuna. If I go out to eat, I always find something that fits in the diet. It's a really flexible program. It's simple to substitute other dishes—all you have to do is stay within the flavor theme. So if I loved what I ate the night before, I'll just make it again the next night.

"For the most part, my family did the program with me, especially the dinners. My older child likes al-most all of the recipes, and my younger one (who's a little more finicky) liked some of them. My husband also has lost some weight on the plan.

"People have definitely noticed my weight loss. My stomach is my problem area, and they tell me it's getting smaller and that my clothes look looser.

"But my absolute favorite thing about the program is the way I feel. I have so much more energy. The sleepy midafternoon feeling has gone away, I have more energy to do things on the weekends, and I find myself staying up later without feeling tired in the morning.

"I would tell anyone to do Dr. Katz's Flavor Point program. The foods are healthful, and you don't sacrifice flavor. And I'm only human. Sometimes I crave something, and I have it. Dr. Katz says, 'If you really, really want something, eat it; otherwise you'll try to make up for the craving in other ways, and it's going to be worse.' I'm definitely going to stick with the program for life." ■

REDUCING SUGAR IN BAKED GOODS

Use the following substitutions for some of the sugar in your recipes.

Nonfat dry milk. The natural sugar (lactose) found in milk sweetens baked goods, although less so than sugar. That's a good thing, because your Flavor Point–trained taste buds will now prefer foods that are less sweet. Replace one-third to one-half of the sugar in your recipes with nonfat dry milk. For instance, if a recipe calls for 1 cup granulated sugar, use ⅔ cup sugar and ⅓ cup dry milk. For examples of using this strategy, see the muffin recipes (starting on page 142), Peach Flat Cake (page 235), Mango-Blueberry Clafoutis (page 253), Chocolate Brownies (page 232), and Oatmeal Chocolate Chip Cookies.

Ground almonds. You can use finely ground almonds to reduce some of the sugar needed in recipes. Experiment with your favorites to see what works best. The slight richness of nuts enhances both the taste and texture of baked goods. For examples, see Peach Flat Cake, Mango-Blueberry Clafoutis, Chocolate Brownies, and Oatmeal Chocolate Chip Cookies.

Unsweetened applesauce or apple butter. Although either applesauce or apple butter is generally used to replace butter in baked goods, it also reduces the amount of sugar needed in those recipes (again, you'll need to experiment to determine the right amount of either ingredient for each recipe). This is because apples contain natural fruit sugar, or fructose. They also provide nutrients and soluble fiber not found in sugar! For an example of how to use this strategy, here's a recipe for Oatmeal Chocolate Chip Cookies.

Oatmeal Chocolate Chip Cookies

You won't actually taste the applesauce in these cookies. Using it is just a way to make them lusciously rich while keeping them low in fat. They also provide heart-healthy oils from the almonds, are rich in fiber from the oats, have added calcium from the nonfat dry milk, and contain relatively little added sugar.

MAKES 3 DOZEN COOKIES

$1/2$ cup almonds

$2/3$ cup unsweetened applesauce

$1/3$ cup nonfat dry milk

$1/2$ cup granulated sugar

6 tablespoons Smart Balance spread

1 whole egg + 1 egg white

1 cup rolled oats

$1/2$ cup soft wheat pastry flour*

1 cup Ghirardelli Double Chocolate Chips

1. Preheat the oven (preferably a convection oven) to 350°F. Line baking sheets with ungreased parchment paper.

2. Grind the almonds to a fine powder in a coffee grinder.

3. Place the applesauce, dry milk, sugar, spread, and the egg and egg white in the bowl of an electric mixer and beat well.

4. Add the almonds, oats, and flour and beat until well blended. Stir in the chocolate chips.

5. Spoon the dough onto the baking sheets and bake, in batches if necessary, for 10 to 12 minutes. Let cool.

Per cookie: 81 calories, 4 g fat (1 g sat fat), 2 g protein, 10 g carbohydrate, 1 g fiber; 5 mg cholesterol, 23 mg sodium

*Arrowhead Mills Organic Pastry Flour or any other brand of soft wheat (not whole wheat) flour with fiber is fine. You can also use Hodgson Mill Oat Bran Flour.

REDUCING FAT IN MOST COOKED DISHES

Use the following substitutions in place of saturated fat.

Olive oil. In all of your cooked dishes, replace all of the butter called for with olive oil. Add a spout to your olive oil bottle to easily control the amount you pour.

Fat-free dairy products. In all cooking or baking, use fat-free milk or yogurt in place of regular milk or yogurt.

Broth. When a recipe calls for broth, use fat-free vegetable or chicken broth with no added sugar.

Skinless poultry. Use only skinless poultry (roast chicken is an exception; it's okay to leave the skin on top for presentation!). Use white-meat chicken or turkey except when a long cooking time would dry it out. In those cases, use thighs or drumsticks with the skin removed (have the butcher at the supermarket remove it for you). For ideas on how to cook chicken, check out Honey Curry–Glazed Chicken (page 191) and Carrot Cider–Glazed Chicken (page 180).

Water. Add about 1 tablespoon of water for every 2 teaspoons of olive oil in salad dressing. This will increase the volume of the dressing so it coats the salad with less fat. You used this strategy to make all of the variations of spinach-lentil salad (pages 168–169).

REDUCING FAT IN BAKED GOODS

Use these substitutions for butter.

Smart Balance spread. To eliminate the saturated fat found in butter or the trans fat found in stick margarines, replace the amount of either ingredient called for in a recipe with the same amount of nonhydrogenated tub margarine, such as Smart Balance. The recipe for Peach Flat Cake uses this substitution.

Ground almonds. Finely ground almonds replace fat as well as some of the sugar in baked goods. They create the richness of butter while adding healthful unsaturated fat in place of saturated fat, and, unlike other nuts, they have a mild flavor that can enhance a recipe without overpowering it. You'll need to use some trial and error to learn the right amount of almonds to use, as it will vary from recipe to recipe. The recipes for Oatmeal Chocolate Chip Cookies, Peach Flat Cake, Mango-Blueberry Clafloutis, and Chocolate Brownies use this substitution.

Unsweetened applesauce or apple butter. When making baked goods, you can use applesauce or apple butter to replace not only some of the sugar but also some of the fat, without losing the moisture that fat usually provides. Replace some of the butter you remove from a recipe with some applesauce or apple butter. Experiment to find the right amount. To see this method in action, take a look at the recipe for Oatmeal Chocolate Chip Cookies.

Soft silken tofu. As long as you discard the extra water, plain silken tofu is a great substitute for butter in brownie recipes. You used this strategy when you made Chocolate Brownies.

Mango-Blueberry Clafoutis

These hearty French peasant custards feature a mango flavor. They take a little more time to prepare than some other desserts but are well worth it! Traditional clafoutis is made with cream, eggs, lots of sugar, and sometimes even butter. In this recipe, Catherine has reduced the number of eggs, eliminated the cream and butter, and reduced the sugar significantly by replacing some of it with the natural sugar in nonfat dry milk. The whole grain flour and ground almonds add fiber to boot! The result is a gem of a dessert that is delicious and nutritious.

MAKES 9 SERVINGS

$1^1/_2$ cups fresh mango, finely chopped

$^3/_4$ cup fresh blueberries

2 tablespoons dark rum*

Grated peel of 1 lemon

3 tablespoons granulated sugar

$^3/_4$ cup fat-free milk

2 whole eggs + 1 egg yolk

$^1/_4$ cup nonfat dry milk

1 tablespoon Smart Balance spread, melted

$^1/_4$ cup finely ground almonds

$^2/_3$ cup soft wheat pastry flour[†]

Confectioners' sugar

1. Preheat a convection oven to 350°F.

2. In a small bowl, combine the mango, blueberries, rum, lemon peel, and 1 tablespoon of the sugar and toss to coat. Let stand for 15 minutes, then drain in a colander over a bowl, reserving the juice.

3. Place the milk, eggs and egg yolk, dry milk, spread, reserved fruit juice, and the remaining 2 tablespoons sugar in the bowl of an electric mixer and beat well.

4. Place the almonds in a medium bowl, sift the flour over them, and stir with a fork to blend. Using a wire whisk, gradually stir the batter into the flour mixture (do not overbeat).

5. Divide the fruit among 9 foil tart pans (4$^1/_2$" in diameter) or place on the bottom of a large, round, deep pie pan. Ladle the batter equally over the fruit. Place the pans on a baking sheet and bake for 25 to 30 minutes, or until puffed and golden. Dust with the confectioners' sugar and serve warm.

Per serving: 155 calories, 5 g fat (1 g sat fat), 5 g protein, 22 g carbohydrate, 2 g fiber, 72 mg cholesterol, 55 mg sodium

*We prefer Mount Gay.

[†]Arrowhead Mills Organic Pastry Flour or any other brand of soft wheat (not whole wheat) flour with fiber is fine. You can also use Hodgson Mill Oat Bran Flour.

REDUCING FAT IN SAUCES AND GLAZES

Use the following substitutions.

Fat-free buttermilk. Replace heavy cream or sour cream with fat-free buttermilk in creamy soups and sauces. You used this strategy when you made Chicken in Creamy Dijon Mushroom Sauce (page 184); Apple–Butternut Squash Soup (page 217); Mint, Sweet Pea, and Spinach Soup (page 222); and Pumpkin Soup (page 223).

Dried fruit and/or natural fruit preserves. As long as they have no added sugar or high-fructose corn syrup, you can simmer dried fruits (such as apricots, raisins, cranberries, peaches, or prunes) or preserves with fat-free chicken broth and/or 100% fruit juice and/or wine or dark beer to create a luscious, rich glaze. You don't need to add butter, sugar, syrup, or molasses to achieve the richness of these dishes. You used this strategy when you made Roast Chicken with Currant Wine Glaze and Caramelized Onions (page 188), Cranberry and Sweet Onion Turkey Cutlets (page 197), Apple-Prune Chicken (page 196), and Peach-Coriander Turkey with Oven-Roasted Potatoes and Turnips (page 198).

Honey mixed with mustard and/or unsweetened juice concentrate. You can use this as a marinade to coat shrimp, tuna, or chicken for the grill. Use just enough honey to make the marinade sticky and rich but not enough to overpower the flavor of the dish. You used this strategy when you made Pineapple Shrimp (page 210) and Honey Curry–Glazed Chicken (page 191).

REDUCING FAT IN NUT-CRUSTED FISH OR CHICKEN

Use this substitution.

Kashi TLC Original 7-Grain cracker crumbs. To cut down on the fat and calories found in the nuts needed to thoroughly coat chicken cutlets or fish fillets, replace half the amount of nuts you would normally use with the same amount of ground crackers (grind them finely in a coffee grinder or small food processor). They'll add volume without much fat and boost fiber as well. To keep the flavor mild, use only the original plain crackers, not the ranch or honey-sesame flavor. You used this strategy in the Flavor Point plan when you made Poppy Seed–Crusted Salmon (page 208), Pecan-Crusted Chicken (page 192), Pistachio-Crusted Chicken (page 187), and Almond-Crusted Tilapia (page 201).

REDUCING FAT IN STUFFING

Use the following substitution.

Bulgur wheat and Kashi TLC Original 7-Grain cracker crumbs. Packaged bread crumbs and readymade stuffings typically contain trans fat and superfluous flavor enhancers. Eliminate these by using a combination of roughly equal amounts of finely ground Kashi crackers and uncooked bulgur wheat, sautéed with chopped onions and celery and cooked with fat-free chicken broth. This method also adds fiber to your meal. The recipes for Roast Chicken with Pecan Stuffing and Portobello Mushrooms with Walnut Stuffing (page 220) use this strategy.

Roast Chicken with Pecan Stuffing

This delicious dish provides a wonderful taste of Thanksgiving with the added goodness of fiber!

SERVES 6

1	medium roasting chicken
$1/2$	teaspoon salt
	Freshly ground black pepper to taste
1	tablespoon extra-virgin olive oil
1	yellow onion, chopped
2	cloves garlic, chopped
1	cup bulgur wheat (dry)
2	cups fat-free chicken broth

20   Kashi TLC Original 7-Grain Crackers

$^1/_2$ cup chopped pecans

2   stalks celery, chopped

1   tablespoon fresh thyme or 1 teaspoon dried

1   teaspoon ground paprika

1. Preheat the oven to 375°F. Rinse the chicken and pat dry. Remove all of the bottom skin and as much of the skin on the sides as you can with kitchen scissors, leaving only the skin on top. Lightly season the cavity with the salt (use no more than $^1/_4$ teaspoon) and pepper and place the chicken in a roasting pan.

2. Heat the oil in a heavy skillet. Add the onion and garlic and cook for about 5 minutes, or until the onion is softened.

3. Add the bulgur and cook, stirring, for 1 to 2 minutes. Add $1^3/_4$ cups of the broth and cook for 8 to 10 minutes, or until the bulgur is cooked, adding more broth if necessary.

4. Meanwhile, grind the crackers in a coffee grinder or small food processor. Add the cracker crumbs, pecans, celery, thyme, and the remaining $^1/_4$ teaspoon salt to the skillet and stir to combine.

5. Fill the chicken cavity with the stuffing, spray briefly with olive oil spray, and sprinkle with the paprika. Bake for 1 hour.

Per serving: 444 calories, 19 g fat (3 g sat fat), 41 g protein, 27 g carbohydrate, 7 g fiber, 108 mg cholesterol, 444 mg sodium

REDUCING FAT IN BREADING

Use the following substitution.

Nature's Path Organic Heritage Flakes and Kashi TLC Original 7-Grain cracker crumbs. To create crispy breading for fried chicken or fish without the fat, replace commercial coating mixes (which typically contain no fiber and include flavor enhancers and additives, salt and sugar, and often, partially hydrogenated oils) with a mixture of finely ground

Kashi crackers and ground or crushed Nature's Path Heritage Flakes cereal. To see how to use this strategy, check out the following recipe for chicken tenders.

Crispy Chicken Tenders

Crispy on the outside and tender on the inside, this dish is also rich in fiber and lean protein. Serve the chicken with Alexia Yukon Gold julienne fries (a 1-pound bag for 4 servings) and a tossed salad. You can also use this recipe to make fish tenders. Just replace the chicken with 1 pound of cod loin (choose captain's cut), cut into long strips.

SERVES 4

1	pound chicken cutlets
$^1/_2$	teaspoon salt
1	cup Nature's Path Heritage Flakes
25	Kashi TLC Original 7-Grain Crackers
1	tablespoon extra-virgin olive oil

1. Preheat the oven to 425°F. Rinse the chicken and pat dry. Cut into long strips and salt lightly (use no more than $^1/_8$ teaspoon of the salt).

2. Place the cereal, crackers, and the remaining salt in a food processor and process into crumbs.

3. On a flat plate, dredge the chicken in the crumbs, coating all sides well and pressing the crumbs firmly into the flesh. Set aside.

4. Heat the oil in a large, ovenproof nonstick skillet. Add the chicken and sear over medium-high heat for 2 to 3 minutes on each side, or until browned.

5. Transfer the skillet to the oven and bake for 5 minutes, or until crisp and golden.

Per serving: 251 calories, 8 g fat (1 g sat fat), 26 g protein, 19 g carbohydrate, 3 g fiber, 63 mg cholesterol, 490 mg sodium

REDUCING FAT IN CHOCOLATE FROSTING

Use these substitutions.

Fat-free milk, nonfat dry milk, and bittersweet chocolate. Most chocolate frosting is made with either heavy cream or hydrogenated oil (trans fat) and flavor enhancers, including salt, sugar, and high-fructose corn syrup. You can do better! Make rich chocolate frosting using fat-free milk, dry milk, and bittersweet chocolate. The following will yield enough frosting for 20 cupcakes. Spread it on Banana–Chocolate Chip Soft Wheat Muffins (page 143). Kids love them with this frosting.

- Combine ⅓ cup fat-free milk and 1 tablespoon dry milk in a small saucepan and bring to a boil.
- Remove from the heat and stir in 3 ounces bittersweet chocolate (six sections of a Ghirardelli baking bar) until smooth.
- Let cool for at least 15 minutes, until the frosting thickens to a perfect creamy consistency.

Instead of using sugary sprinkles on top, try this tip. Slice the stems off large fresh strawberries and place one on top of each cupcake with the pointed end up. Insert a 4-inch decorative wooden pick through each strawberry and into the cupcake. The cupcakes will look as if they're wearing festive party hats!

INCREASING FIBER IN COOKIES AND CAKES

Use the following substitution.

Pastry flour. Replace all of the white flour called for in the recipe with organic pastry flour (such as Arrowhead Mills). Don't confuse this type of soft wheat flour with whole wheat flour, which yields too strong a flavor in cookies and cakes. You can also use oat bran flour (such as Hodgson Mill), which is just as mild tasting and high in fiber as the pastry flour.

ADDING FIBER TO MEAT LOAF AND TURKEY BURGERS

Use this substitution.

Flax meal and Kashi TLC Original 7-Grain cracker crumbs. Use these to replace the processed bread crumbs called for in recipes for meat loaf and burgers. You'll need to use some trial and error to find which amount is best for your recipes. In addition to adding fiber, the flax meal provides omega-3 essential fatty acids, which are often deficient even in well-balanced diets. See the following recipe for Turkey Meat Loaf for inspiration.

Turkey Meat Loaf

This is the best meat loaf ever, and the flax meal makes it even better by providing health-promoting omega-3 fatty acids. Serve with corn on the cob and a tossed salad. Since it serves 8, you can use the leftovers to make great sandwiches for the kids' lunches!

SERVES 8

30	Kashi TLC Original 7-Grain Crackers
$2^{1}/_{2}$	pounds lean or extra-lean ground turkey*
$^{1}/_{4}$	cup flax meal
2	egg whites
1	cup mild salsa†
2	cloves garlic, finely chopped
1	small onion, finely chopped
1	cup torn baby spinach
$^{3}/_{4}$	teaspoon salt
	Freshly ground black pepper to taste

1. Preheat the oven to 325°F. Lightly coat a large baking pan with olive oil spray.

2. Grind the crackers in a coffee grinder or small food processor.

3. In a large bowl, combine the cracker crumbs, turkey, flax meal, egg whites,

salsa, garlic, onion, spinach, salt, and pepper. Mix well until the mixture is firm and holds together when shaped.

4. Place in the baking pan and shape into a loaf. Bake for approximately $1^1/_2$ hours. Discard any fat or juices before serving.

Per serving: 222 calories, 4 g fat (0 g sat fat), 38 g protein, 10 g carbohydrate, 2 g fiber, 56 mg cholesterol, 455 mg sodium

*Check the label to be sure it's breast meat only, with no skin. Look for Jennie-O brand if it's available at your supermarket.

†See the appendix for recommended brands.

ADDITIONAL ADVICE FOR A LIFETIME OF EATING

To maintain the Flavor Point lifestyle, keep the following advice front and center at all times.

- Always aim for variety over time, not variety all the time. Limit the variety of flavors in any given meal or snack, and never cruise from snack to snack.
- Use daily food patterns as a lifelong adaptation of flavor themes. For example, limit your morning food choices on most days to cereal grains, fruits, and dairy foods, and don't mix in meats, cheese, or salty items. Do the opposite for lunch and afternoon snacks: Have salty and savory items, such as vegetables, lean meats, beans, and nuts, but no sweets. For a sense of closure, end lunch with a hot beverage rather than dessert. At dinner, use a single sauce, spread, or dressing or variations on a single theme, such as citrus marinade for fish and citrus vinaigrette on salad.
- Don't add salt to sweet baked goods. We're all used to putting salt into items such as homemade cookies, brownies, cakes, and muffins, if only out of habit. You know what? Brownies, cookies, cakes, and muffins do not need salt! Some may need baking powder in order to rise, but

most do not need baking soda, which is high in sodium. Break yourself of these habits, and you'll reach the Flavor Point more easily.

- Don't add sugar to salty foods. This is less of a problem in home cooking than in processed foods, but many recipes call for unnecessary sugar, molasses, or corn syrup. Try your recipes without these ingredients and see if they work. On the other hand, if a dish is supposed to be fruity, use either dried, fresh, or concentrated fruit and/or 100% fruit juice or juice concentrate. This way, even when you add sugar, you're adding it in its unprocessed natural state in the company of appetite-suppressing fiber.

- In your home, keep nutritious foods (such as fresh fruit) on display all the time. Keep any addictive foods concealed.

- Always serve less of any dish on a plate than you think you (or family members) will want. Keep more available, but keep it out of sight and serve it only upon request.

- Invest in small plates, bowls, cups, and glasses. The average diameter of a dinner plate in the United States has increased by 40 percent since World War II! When you place a normal portion of food on a huge plate, it tricks your brain into thinking you're eating a small amount, which makes you want more.

- On any given day, serve only one kind of dessert. You may break that rule 3 days a year, but no more.

- Serve soups, stews, fizzy beverages (4 ounces of 100% fruit juice mixed with 6 ounces of seltzer water), and smoothies (see pages 150–153) whenever possible to get the benefit of relatively few calories distributed in a large, filling volume.

- Don't buy products that contain trans fat (partially hydrogenated oil).

- Don't buy products that contain high-fructose corn syrup (added sugar).

- Choose products with short ingredient lists.

- Avoid all-you-can-eat buffets.

- Drink water instead of soda and minimize your consumption of artificial sweeteners.

- Don't use more than one sauce, dressing, or spread at any given meal, if possible, and *never* exceed two. In other words, if your pasta sauce has olive oil in it, use olive oil and not butter on your bread. If your chicken has a marinade, use the same marinade with the accompanying grains and vegetables.
- Always start your dinner with a mixed green salad. Salads are nutritious, filling, and low in calories. Use a simple vinaigrette or a dressing that resembles the sauce used for the entrée. For example, squeeze a little lemon in your dressing if you're having a lemon-flavored entrée or add chopped fresh basil to the salad if your entrée includes basil.

BON APPÉTIT

Eating well—for good health and permanent weight control—is, to say the least, challenging in the modern world. You can do it with the right approach and the right knowledge, skills, and strategies. Now you have all of those tools. I believe in you! I hope that by now, you believe in yourself, too!

You have learned how appetite has been controlling you, and you have learned how to control appetite at its source. You have learned how the food industry has been manipulating you into eating more than you should, and you have learned how to choose foods so that you feel fully satisfied with less. You have learned to master the Flavor Point!

With this knowledge, you don't need me anymore. You don't need those training wheels, but if you don't think you're quite ready for solo cruising, that's fine. Back up a bit. Repeat some or all of the meal plan.

You can keep the training wheels for as long as you want, but when you feel confident, take them off and pedal away. I want you to have the kind of relationship with food that my patients, the testers of the Flavor Point Diet, and my family and I have. When we sit down to dinner, we feel relaxed. We take pleasure in the unique flavors of the meal, and we feel fulfilled at the meal's end. I want you to apply the Flavor Point principles for the rest of your life so you never need to worry about your weight again. You can cruise past the challenges of confusing food labels, misleading advertisements, and fast-food bargains. You can reconcile the pleasure of good food with the deep gratification of good health.

I wish you and your family a lifetime of good health and good times. *Bon appétit!*

SUGGESTED BRANDS AND PRODUCTS

Although not comprehensive, this guide to brands and products at the supermarket should help speed you along to the Flavor Point. In compiling the guide, I stuck with winners we know and use, which means I probably left out some wonderful products. If you know and love a product and feel confident, based on your label-reading skills, that it fits into the Flavor Point Diet, by all means continue to use it.

I also limited the guide to brands that are nationally available. If you know of a local brand that's a favorite and meets Flavor Point standards, go for it!

BAKING NEEDS

The nutritional quality and Flavor Point–friendliness of your baked goods depends entirely on what you put into them! The ingredients you choose make all the difference. Put winning ingredients like these in, and you'll get winning results every time.

- Arrowhead Mills whole grain flours, particularly organic pastry flour, for cakes and cookies
- Bob's Red Mill whole grain flours
- Flax meal or whole flaxseeds (any brand)

- Hodgson Mill whole grain flours, particularly oat bran
- King Arthur whole wheat flour
- Ghirardelli Double Chocolate Chips
- Hershey's Unsweetened Cocoa

BREADS

Flavor Point principle: Always choose whole grain bread. Avoid breads with added sugar and fat. Look for low-salt varieties and insist on at least 2 grams of fiber per 100 calories.

- Alvarado Street Bakery Sprouted Rye Seed or any other whole grain variety
- The Baker 9-Grain Whole Wheat or any other whole grain variety
- Country Kitchen Baker: any variety of whole grain bread
- Joseph's Lavash Roll-Ups, Oat Bran Pitas, Whole Wheat Pitas, Whole Wheat Tortillas
- Natural Ovens Right Wheat, 100% Whole Grain, Multigrain, or any other whole grain variety
- Tumaro Gourmet Tortillas
- Vermont Bread Company Whole Wheat, Sprouted Whole Wheat, Soft Whole Wheat, or any other whole grain variety

CANNED OR JARRED GOODS

This is potentially a very large category. Fortunately, there's no need to go over everything here because you already know the general Flavor Point principles and can rely on them to navigate among the many choices you encounter when you shop. In particular, avoid items with clashing flavors and loads of sugar, salt, or added oil. To help you along, here are just a few specific examples of winning entries in this category.

- Canned chicken, tuna, or salmon in water
- Canned fruit in fruit juice
- Canned soup made from broth, with less than 500 milligrams of sodium per serving
- Unsweetened applesauce

CEREAL BARS

Apply the same criteria to cereal bars that you apply to cereals, and you'll see that very few make the Flavor Point cut.

- Barbara's Bakery Puffins Cereal & Milk Bars
- Health Valley Café Creations, granola bars, fruit-filled cereal bars
- Kashi Chewy Granola Bars
- Nature's Choice Multigrain Cereal
- Nature's Path Granola Bars
- Odwalla Nourishing Food Bars

CEREALS

Although cereal can and should be a wonderfully healthful food, the ones you find in every supermarket run the gamut from great to ghastly. Some are simply candy disguised as a breakfast food! This is especially true of cereals peddled to children. Don't buy cereals that don't list a whole grain as the first item on the ingredient list. Avoid cereals with partially hydrogenated oils and with more than 1.5 milligrams of sodium for every calorie; these are salty cereals! Look for cereals with at least 2, and preferably 3, grams of fiber per 100 calories.

- Arrowhead Mills cereals
- Barbara's Bakery cereals, especially Puffins (for kids)
- Cascadian Farm cereals

- Erewhon: cereals, especially Crispy Brown Rice (used in the Peanut Katz Flax Crisps recipe)
- Familia Swiss Muesli
- Health Valley cereals, especially Organic Blue Corn Flakes and Organic Healthy Fiber Multigrain Flakes
- Hodgson Mill hot cereals
- Kashi Heart to Heart, GoLean, Good Friends, Organic Promise Autumn Wheat
- Kretschmer Wheat Germ
- Nature's Path hot and cold cereals, especially FlaxPlus Flakes, Organic Heritage Flakes, Organic Multigrain Oat Bran Flakes, and Optimum; Envirokids (for kids)
- New Morning Organic Oatios, Organic Fruit-e-O's, Corn Flakes (for kids)
- Peace Cereal cereals
- Post Shredded Wheat 'N Bran
- Quaker hot cereals

CHIPS AND CRACKERS

As with breads, chips and crackers can be a good source of fiber and whole grain goodness, or they can be delivery systems for an overload of sugar, salt, and trans fat! The list below will guide you to snacks worthy of the Flavor Point seal of approval!

- Ak-Mak 100% Whole Wheat Sesame Crackers
- Cape Cod Reduced-Fat Potato Chips
- GeniSoy Deep Sea Salt Soy Crisps
- Guiltless Gourmet baked chips
- Kashi TLC Original 7-Grain Crackers
- Old London Whole Wheat Melba Toasts and Whole Wheat Melba Snacks
- Snyder's of Hanover Oat Bran or Honey Wheat Sticks
- Stacy's Simply Naked Baked Pita Chips
- Wasa Light Rye or Hearty Rye Crispbreads

COOKIES

Cookies are a treat. Even when indulging, however, you can make smarter choices. What makes a cookie bad? Trans fat, excess sugar, excess salt, and often, all of these and then some! What makes a cookie good? Great taste and a wholesome economy of ingredients with nothing inside that doesn't belong there.

- Barbara's Bakery Whole Wheat Fig Bars, Snackimals, Organic Go-Go Grahams
- Barry's Bakery French Twists
- Health Valley cookies
- Nature's Promise cookies
- Newman's Own Organics Fig Newmans, Newman-O's

DAIRY PRODUCTS

Dairy foods are great sources of calcium and high-quality protein. They can also contain unwelcome saturated fat and unnecessary quantities of salt. Where is the Flavor Point amidst the curds and whey? Right this way. Limit types with 8 or more grams of fat per ounce.

CHEESE

- Low-fat, part-skim, or fat-free varieties, including ricotta, mozzarella, string cheese, feta cheese, and cottage cheese
- Freshly grated Parmesan

COFFEE CREAMERS

- Undiluted nonfat dry milk; avoid all other creamers

MILK

- Fat-free (skim) milk
- Soymilk and low-fat soymilk (as nondairy alternatives)
- Farmland Dairies Skim Plus
- Hood Simply Smart Fat-Free Milk
- Stonyfield Farm Fat-Free Organic Milk

YOGURT AND PUDDINGS

- Fat-free varieties with active cultures
- Stonyfield Farm all-natural fat-free yogurt (all flavors), O'Soy, Organic Squeezers Portable Lowfat Yogurt (especially for kids) and all-natural organic juice smoothies
- Kozy Shack puddings

DIPS AND SALSA

Dips run the gamut from delicious, nutritious accompaniments to your favorite (Flavor Point–friendly!) chips or crackers to concoctions that probably should be marked with a skull and crossbones. Although not quite as deadly as the dips, some salsas violate Flavor Point rules by adding sugar, salt, and even unnecessary oil. We recommend the following.

- EatSmart Tres Bean Dip
- Green Mountain Gringo salsas
- Guiltless Gourmet salsas and bean dips
- Miguel's Stowe Away salsas
- Muir Glen Organic salsas
- Newman's Own salsas
- Seeds of Change salsa
- Walnut Acres salsa

DRESSINGS

Balsamic vinaigrette is a dressing. So are blue cheese and ranch. Nutritionally, these dressings differ as much as night does from day. Pour the wrong dressing over your so-called salad, and you may consume more calories than you would if you ate a hamburger and french fries! When you dress your salads and other side dishes well, you get wonderful, Flavor Point–friendly taste without clashing flavors. What is the well-dressed, Flavor Point–friendly salad wearing these days? Follow these recommendations.

- Apple cider vinegar
- Avocado oil
- Balsamic vinegar
- Canola oil
- Corn oil
- Extra-virgin olive oil
- Flaxseed oil
- Grapeseed oil
- Red wine vinegar
- Rice wine vinegar
- Walnut oil
- White wine vinegar
- Annie's Naturals dressings
- Brianna's Real French Vinaigrette
- Cains dressings
- Newman's Own Light Italian Dressing and Olive Oil & Vinegar
- Rao's Homemade Red Wine Vinaigrette

ETHNIC FOODS

Although I didn't develop the Flavor Point Diet with any particular ethnic diet in mind, you can certainly adapt it to fit whatever type of food and flavorings you like. The principles apply to any cuisine, from French and

Chinese to Mexican and Italian. Here are several popular categories of commercial ethnic foods that meet Flavor Point criteria.

ASIAN

- Light soy sauce
- Light teriyaki sauce

ITALIAN

- Mancini Roasted Peppers

MIDDLE EASTERN

- Athenos hummus
- Casbah falafel
- Near East hummus and falafel
- Joseph's hummus, tahini, Lavash Roll-Ups, Whole Wheat Pitas
- Telma Falafel Mix

SPANISH

- Goya Recaito, Sofrito, and Sazón seasonings

TEX-MEX

- Joseph's Fat-Free or Low-Fat Tortillas
- Old El Paso fat-free refried beans and bean dips

FROZEN ENTRÉES AND SIDE DISHES

In general, I recommend that you avoid packaged dinners. Even the best of them are very high in sodium. That said, I try never to make perfect the enemy of good, so if, in a pinch, you need to rely on someone else's cooking, use these winners.

- Alexia Oven Fries
- Amy's meals
- Cedarlane meals
- Dr. Praeger's veggie burgers
- Franklin Farms Veggiburgers
- Gardenburger Meals
- Linda McCartney meals
- Moosewood meals
- Nature's Promise meals
- Seeds of Change Organic Frozen Entrées
- Weight Watchers Smart Ones

JUICES AND DRINKS

Your best bet is to drink water instead of juice or other flavored beverages. When you do make other choices, choose wisely! Steer clear of "coolers," "drinks," and "punches." These beverages are generally loaded with added sugar and a big batch of chemicals. I encourage you to drink no soda at all, but, if you must, choose diet. Unless you are physically active for hours on end (as in riding in the Tour de France), you don't need sports drinks! Water is always your best bet.

- Bolthouse Farms 100% fruit smoothies
- Dole 100% Pineapple Juice
- Juicy Juice 100% fruit juices
- Honest T teas
- Martinelli 100% fruit juices
- Nantucket Nectars 100% fruit juices
- Sunsweet 100% fruit juices
- Very Fine Fruit$_2$O
- Welch's 100% fruit juices

MARGARINE

When margarine is good for you, it's very, very good—and when it's bad, it's horrid! Stick margarines are comprised mostly of harmful trans fat that will raise your cholesterol and damage your blood vessels, even more than butter will. Some margarines, on the other hand, are actually designed to lower your cholesterol and improve your heart health. They taste good, too, meeting Flavor Point standards.

- Benecol Spread
- Promise Buttery Spread
- Smart Balance Spread
- Take Control 35% Vegetable Oil Spread

PANCAKES AND WAFFLES

Pancakes and waffles can provide plenty of fiber and whole grain goodness or serve as delivery systems for sugar, salt, and trans fat. The list below will help you choose Flavor Point–approved products.

- Arrowhead Mills Multigrain Pancake and Waffle Mix
- Kashi GoLean waffles
- Van's All-Natural waffles

PASTA AND SAUCES

Get used to hearty whole grain pastas and stick with simple sauces that don't mix together too many flavors.

- Annie's Organic Whole Wheat Shells and Cheddar (for kids)
- Barilla Plus whole grain pastas

- Bertolli Tomato & Basil Sauce
- Buitoni basil pesto spread
- Classico Tomato and Basil Sauce
- Dececco whole wheat pastas
- Hodgson Mill organic whole wheat pastas with flaxseed and other whole grain varieties
- Muir Glen organic pasta sauces and tomatoes
- Rao's Homemade Marinara Sauce

PEANUT BUTTER

All you really need to make peanut butter is . . . peanuts! A bit of salt is a reasonable addition. But sugar? Trans fat? Come on! Choosy parents do not choose to feed their kids combinations of sugar, salt, and partially hydrogenated oil. Avoid "nutty" choices and follow these guidelines.

- Arrowhead Mills Oganic Creamy Valencia Peanut Butter
- Maple Grove Farms Natural Peanut Butter
- Smucker's No Salt Added Natural Peanut Butter
- Teddy's Old-Fashioned Unsalted Peanut Butter
- Trader Joe's All-Natural Peanut Butter

STUFFINGS AND BREAD CRUMBS

In some food categories, all of the commercial choices are bad, and this is one of them. The good news: You can make your own stuffing bread and bread crumbs by crumbling whole grain bread or grinding Kashi TLC Original 7-Grain Crackers. There are terrific Flavor Point tips for making stuffing in Chapter 6, so take this one into your own hands and steer clear of the many commercial losers.

SWEET TOPPINGS

Whenever possible, look for these suggestions to sweeten your desserts.

- 100% maple syrup
- Pure, natural honey
- Hero, Fiordifrutta, Polaner All Fruit, St. Dalfour, Sorrell Ridge preserves

SELECTED BIBLIOGRAPHY

Almiron-Roig E, Chen Y, Drewnowski A. 2003. "Liquid calories and the failure of satiety: How good is the evidence?" *Obes Rev* 4:201–12.

American College of Preventive Medicine Position Statement. *"Diet in the prevention and control of obesity, insulin resistance, and type II diabetes."* www.acpm.org/2002-057(F).htm.

Anderson GH, Moore SE. 2004. "Dietary proteins in the regulation of food intake and body weight in humans." *J Nutr* 134:974S–79S.

Ball SD, Keller KR, Moyer-Mileur LJ, Ding YW, Donaldson D, Jackson WD. 2003. "Prolongation of satiety after low versus moderately high glycemic index meals in obese adolescents." *Pediatrics* 111:488–94.

Baschetti R. "Paleolithic nutrition." 1997. *Eur J Clin Nutr* 51:715–16.

Bell EA, Roe LS, Rolls BJ. 2003. "Sensory-specific satiety is affected more by volume than by energy content of a liquid food." *Physiol Behav* 78:593–600.

Bellisle F. 2003. "Why should we study human food intake behaviour?" *Nutr Metab Cardiovasc Dis* 13:189–93.

Berthoud HR. 2004. "Mind versus metabolism in the control of food intake and energy balance." *Physiol Behav* 81:781–93.

Bjorck I, Elmstahl HL. 2003. "The glycaemic index: Importance of dietary fibre and other food properties." *Proc Nutr Soc* 62:201–6.

Blass EM. 2003. "Biological and environmental determinants of childhood obesity." *Nutr Clin Care* 6:13–19.

Blundell JE, Burley VJ, Cotton JR, Lawton CL. 1993. "Dietary fat and the control of energy intake: Evaluating the effects of fat on meal size and postmeal satiety." *Am J Clin Nutr* 57(5 Suppl):772S–77S.

Blundell JE, Lawton CL, Cotton JR, Macdiarmid JI. 1996. "Control of human appetite: Implications for the intake of dietary fat." *Annu Rev Nutr* 16:285–319.

Blundell JE, MacDiarmid JI. 1997. "Fat as a risk factor for overconsumption: Satiation, satiety, and patterns of eating." *J Am Diet Assoc* 97(7 Suppl):S63–69.

Blundell JE, Stubbs RJ. 1999. "High and low carbohydrate and fat intakes: Limits imposed by appetite and palatability and their implications for energy balance." *Eur J Clin Nutr* 53 Suppl 1:S148–65.

Brand-Miller JC, Holt SH, Pawlak DB, McMillan J. 2002. "Glycemic index and obesity." *Am J Clin Nutr* 76:281S–85S.

Bray GA. 2000. "Afferent signals regulating food intake." *Proc Nutr Soc* 59:373–84.

Critchley HD, Rolls ET. 1996. "Responses of primate taste cortex neurons to the astringent tastant tannic acid." *Chem Senses* 21(2):135–45.

Crovetti R, Porrini M, Santangelo A, Testolin G. 1998. "The influence of thermic effect of food on satiety." *Eur J Clin Nutr* 52:482–88.

Dallman MF, La Fleur SE, Pecoraro NC, Gomez F, Houshyar H, Akana SF. 2004.

"Minireview: Glucocorticoids—food intake, abdominal obesity, and wealthy nations in 2004." *Endocrinology* 145:2633–38.

De Araujo IE, Rolls ET, Kringelbach ML, McGlone F, Phillips N. 2003. "Taste-olfactory convergence, and the representation of the pleasantness of flavour, in the human brain." *Eur J Neurosci* 18(7):2059–68.

De Graaf C, Blom WA, Smeets PA, Stafleu A, Hendriks HF. 2004. "Biomarkers of satiation and satiety." *Am J Clin Nutr* 79:946–61.

De Graaf C, De Jong LS, Lambers AC. 1999. "Palatability affects satiation but not satiety." *Physiol Behav* 66:681–88.

De Graaf C, Schreurs A, Blauw YH. 1993. "Short-term effects of different amounts of sweet and nonsweet carbohydrates on satiety and energy intake." *Physiol Behav* 54:833–43.

DeLorgeril M, Salen P, Martin JL, Monjaud I, Delaye J, Mamelle N. 1999. "Mediterranean diet, traditional risk factors, and the rate of cardiovascular complications after myocardial infarction: Final report of the Lyon Diet Heart Study." *Circulation* 99:779–85.

Drewnowski A. 1998. "Energy density, palatability, and satiety: Implications for weight control." *Nutr Rev* 56:347–53.

———. 2003. "The role of energy density." *Lipids* 38:109–15.

———. 2000. "Sensory control of energy density at different life stages." *Proc Nutr Soc* 59:239–44.

Druce M, Bloom SR. 2003. "Central regulators of food intake." *Curr Opin Clin Nutr Metab Care* 6:361.

Eaton SB, Eaton SB III. 2000. "Paleolithic vs. modern diets—selected pathophysiological implications." *Eur J Nutr* 39:67–70.

Eaton SB, Eaton SB III, Konner M. 1997. "Paleolithic nutrition revisited: A twelve-year retrospective on its nature and implications." *Eur J Clin Nutr* 51:207-16.

Eaton SB, Eaton SB III, Konner M, Shostak M. 1996. "An evolutionary perspective enhances understanding of human nutritional requirements." *J Nutr* 126:1732–40.

Eaton SB, Strassman BI, Nesse RM, Neel JV, Ewald PW, et al. 2002. "Evolutionary health promotion." *Prev Med* 34:109–18.

Ebbeling CB, Leidig MM, Sinclair KB, Hangen JP, Ludwig DS. "A reduced-glycemic load diet in the treatment of adolescent obesity." 2003. *Arch Pediatr Adolesc Med* 157: 773–79.

Flatt JP. 2000. "Macronutrient composition and food selection." *Obes Res* 9 (November) Suppl 4:256S–62S.

Food and Nutrition Board, Institute of Medicine, National Academies of Science. 2002. *Dietary reference intakes for energy, carbohydrate, fiber, fat, fatty acids, cholesterol, protein, and amino acids (macronutrients)*. Washington, D.C.: National Academy Press.

French SA. 2003. "Pricing effects on food choices." *J Nutr* 133:841S–43S.

Gerstein DE, Woodward-Lopez G, Evans AE, Kelsey K, Drewnowski A. 2004. "Clarifying concepts about macronutrients' effects on satiation and satiety." *J Am Diet Assoc* 104:1151–53.

Ginsberg HN, Karmally W, Siddiqui M, Holleran S, Tall AR, Rumsey SC, Deckelbaum RJ, Blaner WS, Ramakrishnan R. 1994. "A dose-response study of the effects of dietary cholesterol on fasting and postprandial lipid and lipoprotein metabolism in healthy young men." *Arterioscler Thromb* 14:576–86.

Golay A, Bobbioni E. 1997. "The role of dietary fat in obesity." *Int J Obes Relat Metab Disord* 21 Suppl 3:S2–11.

Gray RW, French SJ, Robinson TM, Yeomans MR. 2003. "Increasing preload volume with water reduces rated appetite but not food intake in healthy men even with minimum delay between preload and test meal." *Nutr Neurosci* 6:29–37.

Green SM, Blundell JE. 1996. "Effect of fat- and sucrose-containing foods on the size of eating episodes and energy intake in lean dietary restrained and unrestrained females: Potential for causing overconsumption." *Eur J Clin Nutr* 50:625–35.

Green SM, Burley VJ, Blundell JE. 1994. "Effect of fat- and sucrose-containing foods on the size of eating episodes and energy intake in lean males: Potential for causing overconsumption." *Eur J Clin Nutr* 48:547–55.

Green SM, Wales JK, Lawton CL, Blundell JE. 2000. "Comparison of high-fat and high-carbohydrate foods in a meal or snack on short-term fat and energy intakes in obese women." *Br J Nutr* 84:521–30.

Guinard JX, Brun P. 1998. "Sensory-specific satiety: Comparison of taste and texture effects." *Appetite* 31:141–57.

He W, Yasumatsu K, Varadarajan V, Yamada A, Lem J, Ninomiya Y, Margolskee RF, Damak S. 2004. "Umami taste responses are mediated by alpha-transducin and alpha-gustducin." *J Neurosci* 24(35):7674–80.

Hellstrom PM, Geliebter A, Naslund E, Schmidt PT, Yahav EK, Hashim SA, Yeomans MR. 2004. "Peripheral and central signals in the control of eating in normal, obese and binge-eating human subjects." *Br J Nutr* 92 Suppl 1:S47–57.

Hetherington MM. 2002. "The physiological-psychological dichotomy in the study of food intake." *Proc Nutr Soc* 61:497–507.

Holt S, Brand J, Soveny C, Hansky J. 1992. "Relationship of satiety to postprandial glycaemic, insulin and cholecystokinin responses." *Appetite* 18:129–41.

Holt SH, Brand-Miller JC, Petocz P. 1996. "Interrelationships among postprandial satiety, glucose and insulin responses and changes in subsequent food intake." *Eur J Clin Nutr* 50:788–97.

Holt SH, Brand-Miller JC, Stitt PA. 2001. "The effects of equal-energy portions of different breads on blood glucose levels, feelings of fullness and subsequent food intake." *J Am Diet Assoc* 101:767–73.

Holt SH, Miller JC, Petocz P, Farmakalidis E. 1995. "A satiety index of common foods." *Eur J Clin Nutr* 49:675–90.

Howarth NC, Saltzman E, Roberts SB. "Dietary fiber and weight regulation." 2001. *Nutr Rev* 59:129–39.

Hu FB. 2003. "Plant-based foods and prevention of cardiovascular disease: An overview." *Am J Clin Nutr* 78:544S–51S.

Hu FB, Manson JE, Willett WC. 2001. "Types of dietary fat and risk of coronary heart disease: A critical review." *J Am Coll Nutr* 20:5–19.

Hu FB, Stampfer MJ, Rimm EB, Manson JE, Ascherio A, Colditz GA, Rosner BA, Spiegelman D, Speizer FE, Sacks FM, Hennekens CH, Willett WC. 1999. "A prospective study of egg consumption and risk of cardiovascular disease in men and women." *JAMA* 281:1387–94.

Hu FB, Willett WC. 2002. "Optimal diets for prevention of coronary heart disease." *JAMA* 288:2569–78.

Hung T, Sievenpiper JL, Marchie A, Kendall CW, Jenkins DJ. 2003. "Fat versus carbohydrate in insulin resistance, obesity, diabetes and cardiovascular disease." *Curr Opin Clin Nutr Metab Care* 6:165–76.

Jequier E. 2002. "Pathways to obesity." *Int J Obes Relat Metab Disord* 26 Suppl 2:S12–17.

Johnson J, Vickers Z. 1992. "Factors influencing sensory-specific satiety." *Appetite* 19:15–31.

Katz DL. 2005. "Competing dietary claims for weight loss: Finding the forest through truculent trees." *Annu Rev Public Health* 26:61–88.

———. "Diet, sleep-wake cycles, and mood." In Katz DL. 2001. *Nutrition in clinical practice*. Philadelphia: Lippincott Williams & Wilkins. 243–47.

———. "Dietary recommendations for health promotion and disease prevention." In Katz DL. *Nutrition in clinical practice*. Philadelphia: Lippincott Williams & Wilkins. 291–98.

———. "Evolutionary biology, culture, and determinants of dietary behavior." In Katz DL. 2001. *Nutrition in clinical practice*. Philadelphia: Lippincott Williams & Wilkins. 279–90.

———. "Hunger, appetite, taste, and satiety." In Katz DL. 2001. *Nutrition in clinical practice*. Philadelphia: Lippincott Williams & Wilkins. 260–67.

———. 2001. *Nutrition in clinical practice*. Philadelphia: Lippincott Williams & Wilkins.

Katz DL, Evans MA, Nawaz H, Njike VY, Chan W, Comerford BP, Hoxley ML. 2005. "Egg consumption and endothelial function: A randomized controlled crossover trial." *Int J Cardiol* 99:65–70.

Kennedy E. 2004. "Dietary diversity, diet quality, and body weight regulation." *Nutr Rev* 62(7 Pt 2):S78–81.

Kennedy ET, Bowman SA, Spence JT, Freedman M, King J. 2001. "Popular diets: Correlation to health, nutrition, and obesity." *J Am Diet Assoc* 101:411–20.

Key TJ, Schatzkin A, Willett WC, Allen NE, Spencer EA, Travis RC. 2004. "Diet, nutrition and the prevention of cancer." *Public Health Nutr* 7:187–200.

Knopp RH, Retzlaff BM, Walden CE, Dowdy AA, Tsunehara CH, Austin MA, Nguyen T. 1997. "A double-blind, randomized, controlled trial of the effects of two eggs per day in moderately hypercholesterolemic and combined hyperlipidemic subjects taught the NCEP step I diet." *J Am Coll Nutr* 16:551–61.

Knowler WC, Barrett-Connor E, Fowler SE, Hamman RF, Lachin JM, et al. 2002. "Reduction in the incidence of type 2 diabetes with lifestyle intervention or metformin." *N Engl J Med* 346:393–403.

Kritchevsky SB. 2004. "A review of scientific research and recommendations regarding eggs." *J Am Coll Nutr* 23(6 Suppl):596S–600S.

Kritchevsky SB, Kritchevsky D. 2000. "Egg consumption and coronary heart disease: An epidemiologic overview." *J Am Coll Nutr* 19(5 Suppl):549S–555S.

Lang V, Bellisle F, Oppert JM, Craplet C, Bornet FR, Slama G, Guy-Grand B. 1998. "Satiating effect of proteins in healthy subjects: A comparison of egg albumin, casein, gelatin, soy protein, pea protein, and wheat gluten." *Am J Clin Nutr* 67:1197–204.

Leibowitz SF, Alexander JT. 1998. "Hypothalamic serotonin in control of eating behavior, meal size, and body weight." *Biol Psychiat* 44:851–64.

Liu S, Willett WC, Manson JE, Hu FB, Rosner B, Colditz G. 2003. "Relation between changes in intakes of dietary fiber and grain products and changes in weight and development of obesity among middle-aged women." *Am J Clin Nutr* 78:920–27.

Macht M, Simons G. 2000. "Emotions and eating in everyday life." *Appetite* 35:65–71.

Mann NJ. 2004. "Paleolithic nutrition: What can we learn from the past?" *Asia Pac J Clin Nutr* 13(Suppl):S17.

Marmonier C, Chapelot D, Louis-Sylvestre J. 2000. "Effects of macronutrient content and energy density of snacks consumed in a satiety state on the onset of the next meal." *Appetite* 34:161–68.

Mathers JC. 2003. "Nutrition and cancer prevention: Diet-gene interactions." *Proc Nutr Soc* 62:605–10.

McCrory MA, Fuss PJ, McCallum JE, Yao M, Vinken AG, Hays NP, Roberts SB. 1999. "Dietary variety within food groups: Association with energy intake and body fatness in men and women." *Am J Clin Nutr* 69:440–47.

McCrory MA, Suen VM, Roberts SB. 2002. "Biobehavioral influences on energy intake and adult weight gain." *J Nutr* 132:3830S–34S.

McDonald BE. 2004. "The Canadian experience: Why Canada decided against an upper limit for cholesterol." *J Am Coll Nutr* 23(6 Suppl):616S–20S.

McNamara DJ. 2000. "The impact of egg limitations on coronary heart disease risk: Do the numbers add up?" *J Am Coll Nutr* 19(5 Suppl):540S–48S.

Meier U, Gressner AM. 2004. "Endocrine regulation of energy metabolism: Review of pathobiochemical and clinical chemical aspects of leptin, ghrelin, adiponectin, and resistin." *Clin Chem* 50:1511–25.

National Institutes of Health, National Heart, Lung, and Blood Institute, and the North American Association for the Study of Obesity. "The practical guide to identification, evaluation, and treatment of overweight and obesity in adults." www.nhlbi.nih.gov/guidelines/obesity/prctgd_b.pdf

Nestle M, Wing R, Birch L, DiSogra L, Drewnowski A, Middleton S, Sigman-Grant M, Sobal J, Winston M, Economos C. 1998. "Behavioral and social influences on food choice." *Nutr Rev* 56(5 Pt 2):S50–64; discussion S64–74.

O'Keefe JH Jr, Cordain L. 2004. "Cardiovascular disease resulting from a diet and lifestyle at odds with our paleolithic genome: How to become a 21st-century hunter-gatherer." *Mayo Clin Proc* 79:101–8.

Ornish D, Scherwitz LW, Billings JH, Brown SE, Gould KL, et al. 1998. "Intensive lifestyle changes for reversal of coronary heart disease." *JAMA* 280:2001–7.

Phillips SM, Bandini LG, Naumova EN, Cyr H, Colclough S, Dietz WH, Must A. 2004.

"Energy-dense snack food intake in adolescence: Longitudinal relationship to weight and fatness." *Obes Res* 12:461–72.

Poppitt SD, McCormack D, Buffenstein R. 1998. "Short-term effects of macronutrient preloads on appetite and energy intake in lean women." *Physiol Behav* 64:279–85.

Poppitt SD, Prentice AM. 1996. "Energy density and its role in the control of food intake: Evidence from metabolic and community studies." *Appetite* 26:153–74.

Porrini M, Crovetti R, Riso P, Santangelo A, Testolin G. 1995. "Effects of physical and chemical characteristics of food on specific and general satiety." *Physiol Behav* 57:461–8.

Prentice AM, Jebb SA. 2003. "Fast foods, energy density and obesity: A possible mechanistic link." *Obes Rev.* 4:187–94.

Raben A, Agerholm-Larsen L, Flint A, Holst JJ, Astrup A. 2003. "Meals with similar energy densities but rich in protein, fat, carbohydrate, or alcohol have different effects on energy expenditure and substrate metabolism but not on appetite and energy intake." *Am J Clin Nutr* 77:91–100.

Raynor HA, Epstein LH. 2001. "Dietary variety, energy regulation, and obesity." *Psychol Bull* 127:325–41.

Reddy KS, Katan MB. 2004. "Diet, nutrition and the prevention of hypertension and cardiovascular diseases." *Pub Health Nutr* 7:167–86.

Rolls BJ. 1995. "Carbohydrates, fats, and satiety." *Am J Clin Nutr* 61(4 Suppl):960S–67S.

———. 2000. "The role of energy density in the overconsumption of fat." *J Nutr* 130(2S Suppl):268S–71S.

Rolls BJ, Bell EA. 1999. "Intake of fat and carbohydrate: Role of energy density." *Eur J Clin Nutr* 53 Suppl 1:S166–73.

Rolls BJ, Bell EA, Castellanos VH, Chow M, Pelkman CL, Thorwart ML. 1999. "Energy density but not fat content of foods affected energy intake in lean and obese women." *Am J Clin Nutr* 69:863–71.

Rolls BJ, Bell EA, Thorwart ML. 1999. "Water incorporated into a food but not served with a food decreases energy intake in lean women." *Am J Clin Nutr* 70:448–55.

Rolls BJ, Bell EA, Waugh BA. 2000. "Increasing the volume of a food by incorporating air affects satiety in men." *Am J Clin Nutr* 72:361–68.

Rolls BJ, Castellanos VH, Halford JC, Kilara A, Panyam D, Pelkman CL, Smith GP, Thorwart ML. 1998. "Volume of food consumed affects satiety in men." *Am J Clin Nutr* 67:1170–77.

Rolls BJ, Hetherington M, Burley VJ. 1998. "Sensory stimulation and energy density in the development of satiety." *Physiol Behav* 44:727–33.

Rolls BJ, Miller DL. 1997. "Is the low-fat message giving people a license to eat more?" *J Am Coll Nutr* 16:535–43.

Rolls ET. 2004. "Convergence of sensory systems in the orbitofrontal cortex in primates and brain design for emotion." *Anat Rec A Discov Mol Cell Evol Biol.* 281(1):1212–25.

———. 2000. "The representation of umami taste in the taste cortex." *J Nutr* 130(4S Suppl):960S–65S.

———. 2004. "Smell, taste, texture, and temperature multimodal representations in the brain, and their relevance to the control of appetite." *Nutr Rev* 62(11 Pt 2):S193–204; discussion S224–41.

———. 1997. "Taste and olfactory processing in the brain and its relation to the control of eating." *Crit Rev Neurobiol* 11(4):263–87.

Rolls ET, Critchley HD, Browning A, Hernadi I. 1998. "The neurophysiology of taste and olfaction in primates, and umami flavor." *Ann NY Acad Sci* 855(November 30):426–37.

Romon M, Lebel P, Velly C, Marecaux N, Fruchart JC, Dallongeville J. 1999. "Leptin response to carbohydrate or fat meal and association with subsequent satiety and energy intake." *Am J Physiol* 277(5 Pt 1):E855–61.

Sacks FM, Svetkey LP, Vollmer WM, Appel LJ, Bray GA, et al. 2001. "Effects on blood pressure of reduced dietary sodium and the Dietary Approaches to Stop Hypertension (DASH) diet." *N Engl J Med* 344:3–10.

Saris WH. 2003. "Sugars, energy metabolism, and body weight control." *Am J Clin Nutr* 78:850S–57S.

Shepherd R. 1999. "Social determinants of food choice." *Proc Nutr Soc* 58:807–12.

Small CJ, Bloom SR. 2004. "Gut hormones and the control of appetite." *Trends Endoc Metab* 15(6):259–63.

Snoek HM, Huntjens L, Van Gemert LJ, De Graaf C, Weenen H. 2004. "Sensory-specific satiety in obese and normal-weight women." *Am J Clin Nutr* 80:823–31.

Sorensen LB, Moller P, Flint A, Martens M, Raben A. 2003. "Effect of sensory perception of foods on appetite and food intake: A review of studies on humans." *Int J Obes Relat Metab Disord* 27:1152–66.

Stubbs J, Ferres S, Horgan G. "Energy density of foods: Effects on energy intake." 2000. *Crit Rev Food Sci Nutr* 40:481–515.

Stubbs RJ, Johnstone AM, Mazlan N, Mbaiwa SE, Ferris S. 2001. "Effect of altering the variety of sensorially distinct foods, of the same macronutrient content, on food intake and body weight in men." *Eur J Clin Nutr* 55:19–28.

Stubbs RJ, Whybrow S. 2004. "Energy density, diet composition and palatability: Influences on overall food energy intake in humans." *Physiol Behav* 81:755–64.

U.S. Preventive Services Task Force. "Healthy diet counseling." www.ahrq.gov/clinic/uspstf/uspsdiet.htm; accessed March 2005.

Vickers Z. 1999. "Long-term acceptability of limited diets." *Life Support Biosph Sci* 6:29–33.

Vozzo R, Wittert G, Cocchiaro C, Tan WC, Mudge J, Fraser R, Chapman I. 2003. "Similar effects of foods high in protein, carbohydrate and fat on subsequent spontaneous food intake in healthy individuals." *Appetite* 40:101–7.

Wansink B. 2004. "Environmental factors that increase the food intake and consumption volume of unknowing consumers." *Annu Rev Nutr* 24:455–79.

Wardle J. 1987. "Hunger and satiety: A multidimensional assessment of responses to caloric loads." *Physiol Behav* 40:577–82.

Weggemans RM, Zock PL, Katan MB. 2001. "Dietary cholesterol from eggs increases the ratio of total cholesterol to high-density lipoprotein cholesterol in humans: A meta-analysis." *Am J Clin Nutr* 73:885–91.

Westerterp-Plantenga MS. 2001. "Analysis of energy density of food in relation to energy intake regulation in human subjects." *Br J Nutr* 85:351–61.

Westerterp-Plantenga MS, IJedema MJ, Wijckmans-Duijsens NE. 1996. "The role of macronutrient selection in determining patterns of food intake in obese and non-obese women." *Eur J Clin Nutr* 50:580–91.

Westerterp-Plantenga MS, Lejeune MP, Nijs I, Van Ooijen M, Kovacs EM. 2004. "High protein intake sustains weight maintenance after body weight loss in humans." *Int J Obes Relat Metab Disord* 28:57–64.

Westerterp-Plantenga MS, Rolland V, Wilson SA, Westerterp KR. 1999. "Satiety related to 24-hour diet-induced thermogenesis during high protein/carbohydrate vs high fat diets measured in a respiration chamber." *Eur J Clin Nutr* 53:495–502.

Willet WC. 2001. *Eat, drink, and be healthy.* New York: Simon & Schuster Source.

Wylie-Rosett J, Segal-Isaacson CJ, Segal-Isaacson A. 2004. "Carbohydrates and increases in obesity: Does the type of carbohydrate make a difference?" *Obes Res* 12 Suppl 2:124S–29S.

Wynne K, Stanley S, Bloom S. 2004. "The gut and regulation of body weight." *J Clin Endoc Metab* 89:2576–82.

Zhang Y, Hoon MA, Chandrashekar J, Mueller KL, Cook B, Wu D, Zuker CS, Ryba NJ. 2003. "Coding of sweet, bitter, and umami tastes: Different receptor cells sharing similar signaling pathways." *Cell* 2003 112(3):283–84.

INDEX

Underscored page references indicate boxed text.

Chicken with Chocolate Port Wine
    Sauce, 182–83
Chocolate and Banana Grilled Panini, 178
Chocolate Brownies, 232–33
Mint Chocolate Chip Shake, 243
Oatmeal Chocolate Chip Cookies, 251
Pumpkin and Chocolate Grilled Panini,
    178
Strawberries Dipped in Dark Chocolate,
    241
Chocolate Day, 127
Chow Now meals, 70–71
Clafoutis
    Mango-Blueberry Clafoutis, 253–54
Coconut Day, 128
Coconut milk
    Coconut-Pineapple Smoothie, 150
    Coconut Shrimp and Avocado Salad,
        164
    Coconut Thai Chicken, 186–87
    Piña Colada Frozen Dessert, 238
Cod
    Orange Cod, 204
Coffee, 73
Coffee creamers, suggested, 269
Complex carbohydrates, 32, 33
    in Flavor Point Diet, 32
Cooked dishes, reducing fat in, 252
Cookies
    increasing fiber in, 259
    Oatmeal Chocolate Chip Cookies, 251
    Peanut Katz Flax Crisps, 238–39
    suggested brands of, 269
Corn
    Black Bean, Corn, and Tomato Salad,
        165
Crackers, suggested brands of, 65, 268
Cranberries
    Cranberry and Sweet Onion Turkey
        Cutlets, 197
    Cranberry-Banana Soft Wheat Muffins,
        143
    Cranberry-Lentil Mixed Greens Salad
        with Feta and Pecans, 168–69
    Cranberry-Vanilla Soft Ice Cream, 243
Cranberry Day, 80, 112
Cranberry juice
    Cranberry-Banana Smoothie, 150
Cucumbers
    Cucumber, Tomato, Olive, and Red
        Onion Salad, 212
    Peanut-Cucumber Salad, 170
    Poached Salmon with Cucumber-Dill
        Sauce, 207

Currants
    Currant-Lentil Spinach Salad with Feta
        and Walnuts, 168
    Roast Chicken with Currant Wine Glaze
        and Caramelized Onions, 188
Curry powder
    Curry, Lentil, and Spinach Salad with
        Gorgonzola and Walnuts, 169
    Honey Curry-Glazed Chicken, 191

D

Dairy products
    in cooked dishes, 252
    shopping for, 52, 53, 269
Desserts
    Baked Bananas with Rum-Pecan
        Topping, 230
    Baked Cinnamon-Almond Apples,
        231
    Baked Cinnamon Apples, 231
    Baked Cinnamon-Walnut Apples, 231
    Caramelized Pineapple Rings, 234
    Chocolate Brownies, 232–33
    Cranberry-Vanilla Soft Ice Cream, 243
    flavor guidelines for, 247
    limiting variety of, 262
    Mango-Blueberry Clafoutis, 253–54
    Mint Chocolate Chip Shake, 243
    Oatmeal Chocolate Chip Cookies, 251
    Peach Flat Cake, 235
    Peanut Katz Flax Crisps, 238–39
    Piña Colada Frozen Dessert, 238
    Pumpkin Soft Ice Cream, 244
    Raisin-Granola Parfait, 240
    Strawberries Dipped in Dark Chocolate,
        241
    timing of, 48
    Warm Apple Crisp, 242
Dill
    Asparagus and Dill Cheese Omelet, 148–49
    Dill Chicken Salad Sandwich, 177
    Dill Potatoes, 224
    Dill Yogurt Dip, 154
    Poached Salmon with Cucumber-Dill
        Sauce, 207
Dill Day, 111
Dinner(s)
    Flavor-Friendly Alternatives for, 133
    flavor guidelines for, 247
    recipes for
        fish and shellfish, 201–10
        pasta, 215–16

ABOUT THE AUTHORS

David L. Katz, MD, MPH, FACPM, FACP, is an associate professor of public health at the Yale University School of Medicine. He is the director and cofounder of Yale's Prevention Research Center, associate director of nutrition science at the Rudd Center for Food Policy and Obesity at Yale University, and the founder and director of a holistic clinical facility at the Integrative Medicine Center in Derby, Connecticut.

In addition to more than 80 scientific papers and innumerable columns, essays, op-eds, chapters, essays, and newsletters, Dr. Katz has published eight previous books. Among these are several textbooks for health professionals, including *Nutrition in Clinical Practice,* a nutrition textbook that is widely used in medical education, including at the Harvard Medical School.

Dr. Katz lectures on nutrition, health promotion, and disease prevention throughout the United States and abroad and has consulted on these topics to the U.S. Department of Health and Human Services, the U.S. Food and Drug Administration, and the National Governors Association.

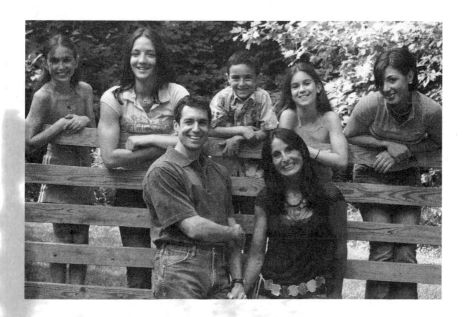

Dr. Katz is a medical contributor for *ABC News,* the nutrition columnist for *O: The Oprah Magazine,* and the author of a syndicated health/nutrition column for the *New York Times.* His expert opinion has been featured in *Business Week, Glamour, Good Housekeeping, Health, Time* magazine, *U.S. News & World Report, Wall Street Journal,* the *Washington Post,* among dozens of other publications.

Catherine S. Katz, PhD, was raised in the south of France and learned the fine art of southern French and North African cooking from her mother and aunt. She came to the United States at age 14, and promptly gained about 25 pounds from her sudden immersion in the "toxic nutritional environment" of the United States. It took her several years to learn all the strategies necessary to compensate for the challenges of that environment and stabilize her weight permanently.

Catherine is a neuroscientist by training, earning her PhD from Princeton University. She has made significant scientific contributions in the area of olfaction (sense of smell) and its links to memory and learning. During recent years, her talents have been devoted to the raising of her five children and raising the standards of gourmet nutrition. Catherine's cooking talents have been featured in *O: The Oprah Magazine, Child, Men's Health, Women's Health & Fitness, Nick Jr.* and several books, as well as in cooking classes for both adults and children at the Silo Cooking School in New Milford, Connecticut, where, among others, Jacques Pepin is an instructor.

Drs. David and Catherine Katz live in Connecticut with their five children: Rebecca (17), Corinda (16), Valerie (11), Natalia (10), and Gabriel (6). The Katz family has been featured in both *Child* and *Men's Health* magazines.